09

SURGERY MCQs AND EMQs

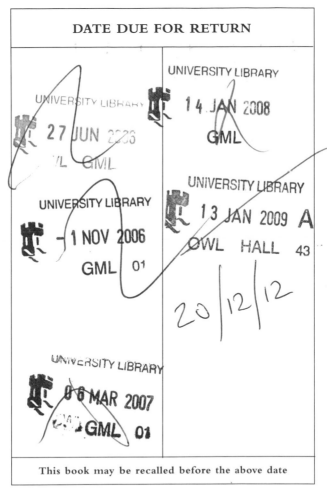
90014

SURGERY MCQs AND EMQs

by
R. W. Parks
MD, FRCSI, FRCS (Ed)
Senior Lecturer/Honorary Consultant Surgeon
Department of Clinical and Surgical Sciences (Surgery)
University of Edinburgh

T. Diamond
BSc, MD, FRCS, FRCSI
Consultant Surgeon
Mater Hospital
Belfast

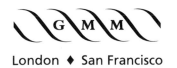

London ♦ San Francisco

www.greenwich-medical.co.uk

© 2003

Greenwich Medical Media Limited
137 Euston Road, London
NW1 2AA

870 Market Street, Ste 720
San Francisco, CA 94102

ISBN 1841101869

First Published 2003

Typeset by Mizpah Publishing Services, Chennai, India
Printed in the UK by the Alden Group, Oxford.

Distributed by Plymbridge Distributors Ltd and
in the USA by JAMCO Distribution

Contents

Section 1 – Multiple Choice Questions (MCQs)

Section 2 – Extended Matching Questions (EMQs)

Preface

This book is designed to be used in conjunction with *Fundamentals of Surgical Practice*, but as explanatory answers are given it may also be used on its own. The content is appropriate for final year medical students and particularly for candidates preparing for the MRCS/AFRCS examination. We recommend that the questions are attempted after studying each topic, but they may also be useful to assess progress and the standard required for success in surgical examinations.

R.W.P.
T.D
April 2003

List of Abbreviations

ABG   Arterial blood gas
ACTH   Adrenocorticotrophic hormone
ADH   Antidiuretic hormone
AFP   Alpha-feto protein
ARDS   Adult respiratory distress syndrome
ASA   American Society of Anesthesiologists

BNH   Benign nodular hyperplasia

CEA   Carcinoembryonic antigen
COAD   Chronic obstructive airways disease
CRF   Corticotropin releasing factor
CSF   Cerebrospinal fluid
CT   Computed tomography
CVP   Central venous pressure

DIC   Disseminated intravascular coagulation
DPL   Diagnostic peritoneal lavage
DVT   Deep vein thrombosis

ECG   Electrocardiogram
EMD   Electromechanical dissociation
ERCP   Endoscopic retrograde cholangio-pancreatogram
ESWL   Extracorporeal shock wave lithotripsy

FNA   Fine-needle aspiration
FNAC   Fine needle aspiration cytology

GCS   Glasgow coma scale/score
GGT   Gamma glutaryl transferase
GI   Gastrointestinal
GORD   Gastro-oesophageal reflux disease

HBV   Hepatitis B virus
HCG   Human chorionic gonadotrophin
HCV   Hepatitis C virus
HIV   Human immunodeficiency virus

IgA   Immunoglobulin A
IgE   Immunoglobulin E
IL   Interleukin
ITP   Idiopathic thrombocytopenic purpura
IV   Intravenous
IVC   Inferior vena cava

LHRH   Luteinising hormone releasing hormone

MEN	Multiple endocrine neoplasia
MODS	Multiple organ dysfunction syndrome
MRSA	Methicillin-resistant staphylococcus aureus
MSH	Melanocyte stimulating hormone
NdYAG	Neodynium yttrium aluminium garnet
NG	Nasogastric
NIDDM	Non-insulin dependent diabetes mellitus
OGD	Oesophago-gastro-duodenoscopy
OPSI	Overwhelming post-splenectomy infection
PAF	Platelet activating factor
PDGF	Platelet-derived growth factor
PEEP	Positive end-expiratory pressure
PEG	Percutaneous gastrostomy
PSA	Prostate specific antigen
PSA	Pleomorphic salivary adenoma
PUJ	Pelvi-ureteric junction
RBC	Red blood cell
SIRS	Systemic inflammatory response syndrome
TCC	Transitional cell carcinoma
TNF	Tumour necrosis factor
TOF	Tracheo-oesophageal fistula
TPN	Total parenteral nutrition
TSH	Thyroid stimulating hormone
VACTERL	Vertebral, anorectal, cardiac, TOF and esophageal atresia, renal and limb
VUR	Vesico-ureteric reflux
WBC	White blood cell
WHO	World Health Organisation

Section 1

Multiple Choice Questions (MCQs)

Q 1. **The American Society of Anesthesiologists (ASA) classification of fitness of patients for surgery includes the following**

   A. ASA 1 where there is no organic, physiological, biochemical or psychiatric disturbance
   B. ASA 3 where there is mild to moderate systemic disturbance which does not limit normal activity
   C. ASA 4 where there are severe life-threatening systemic disorders
   D. ASA 5 where the patient is moribund with little chance of recovery
   E. ASA E where the letter E after a particular classification denotes an emergency operation

Q 2. **Concerning the risk of myocardial infarction during or following surgery**

   A. Infarction <3 months prior to surgery increases the risk by 30%
   B. Infarction >6 months prior to surgery increases the risk by 6%
   C. The risk is 5–10% when there is no previous history of infarction
   D. Elective surgery should not be performed within 6 months of a myocardial infarction
   E. Gastrointestinal endoscopy should not be performed within 6 months of a myocardial infarction

Q 3. **Hypertension**

   A. Is defined by the World Health Organisation as a systolic blood pressure >160 mmHg and/or a diastolic blood pressure >105 mmHg
   B. Is present in approximately 25% of adult patients
   C. Is a contraindication to elective surgery if the diastolic pressure exceeds 115 mmHg

D. Should be treated with intravenous beta-blockers or glyceryl T
trinitrate if emergency surgery is necessary
E. Treatment should be discontinued 2 weeks before elective F
surgery

**Q 4. The following drugs should be discontinued prior to
surgery**

A. Prednisolone F
B. Progesterone-only oral contraceptive pill T
C. Aspirin F
D. Propranolol F
E. Warfarin T

**Q 5. The following investigations are appropriate prior to
surgery**

A. An ECG in all patients >30 years F
B. A chest X-ray on all patients >40 years F
C. A biochemical screen (block) on all patients >30 years F
undergoing major surgery
D. A haematocrit on all female patients F
E. A coagulation screen in all patients with obstructive T
jaundice

Q 6. In a diabetic patient undergoing surgery

A. The dose of depot insulin should be halved on the day prior to T
surgery and supplemented with soluble insulin later in the day
B. Half the morning dose of insulin should be given on the day F
of surgery
C. An intravenous infusion of 5% dextrose is erected on the F
morning of surgery
D. Insulin requirements may increase after major surgery
E. The majority of diabetic patients undergoing surgery have
insulin-dependent (Type I) diabetes

**Q 7. The following statements concerning prophylaxis of
thrombo-embolic disease are true**

A. An appropriate regimen involves enoxaparin 20 mg bd, given
subcutaneously

B. Clinically significant thromboembolism occurs in approximately 1% of patients undergoing major surgery

C. Mechanical measures contribute significantly to reduce the incidence of thromboembolism

D. Dextran 70 is widely used to reduce the incidence of postoperative deep vein thrombosis

E. Age >35 years, obesity and malignancy are all significant risk factors for the development of deep vein thrombosis

Q 1. The following are intravenous induction anaesthetic agents

   A. Propofol   T

   B. Etomidate   T

   C. Sevoflurane   F

   D. Thiopentone   T

   E. Halothane

Q 2. The following are depolarising neuromuscular blocking drugs

   A. Suxamethonium   T

   B. Atracurium   F

   C. Vecuronium   F

   D. Pancuronium   F

   E. Atracurium   F

Q 3. The following statements concerning opioid analgesics are true

   A. Morphine is a synthetic alkaloid   F

   B. Morphine may be administered orally, intravenously, intramuscularly, subcutaneously and via the epidural (neuraxial) route   T

   C. Papavertum contains a mixture of morphine, pethidine and papaverine   F

   D. Fentanyl is a synthetic derivative of morphine

   E. Fentanyl causes significant cardiovascular instability   F

Q 4. The following are correct contents of common crystalloid solutions

   A. NaCl 0.9% contains 154 mmol of sodium per litre   T

   B. NaCl 0.9% contains 72 mmol of chloride per litre   F

C. Glucose 5% contains 20 mmol of potassium per litre   F

D. Hartmann's contains 40 mmol of potassium per litre   F

E. Hartmann's contains 150 kCal per litre   F

Q 5. The following are significant advantages of regional anaesthesia

A. Avoidance of unconsciousness   T

B. Absence of respiratory depression   T

C. Sympathetic blockade   F

D. Blockade of motor function   F

E. Avoidance of Hypotension   F

Q 6. Local anaesthesia

A. Only affects sensory nerve fibres   F

B. Is very effective for incision and drainage of cutaneous abscesses   F

C. Must be injected into the tissues to become effective   F

D. In high doses can cause convulsions and bradycardia   T

E. May not be used in the region of an end-artery   T

Q 7. In general anaesthesia

A. Pulse oximetry is used routinely to record the heart rate and oxygen saturation   T

B. Patients require mechanical ventilation for the operative period   F

C. Preoperative starvation ensures that the stomach is empty   F

D. Bradycardia is treated with neostigmine   F

E. Opioids do not cause direct myocardial depression   T

Postoperative Management

Questions

Q 1. **Complications of blood transfusion are**

  A. Urticaria   T
  B. Hypokalaemia   F
  C. Hepatitis C   T
  D. ARDS   T
  E. Jaundice   T

Q 2. **Atelectasis**

  A. May impair gas exchange   T
  B. May predispose to chest infection   T
  C. Can be prevented by prophylactic treatment with antibiotics   F
  D. Is a common cause of an early postoperative fever   F
  E. May necessitate fibreoptic bronchoscopy to extract mucus plugs   T

Q 3. **Postoperative fluid management of the surgical patient should**

  A. Include administration of 40–60 mmol of potassium in the first 24 h   F
  B. Account for insensible losses of up to 1500 ml if the patient is septic   F
  C. Include packed red blood cells if the haematocrit falls below 40%   F
  D. Aim to provide at least 1000 calories for the first three postoperative days   F
  E. Be increased if the central venous pressure falls below 8 cm H_2O F

Q 4. **With regard to postoperative complications**

  A. The most common site of intra-abdominal abscess formation is in the pelvis   F

B. Secondary haemorrhage is often associated with diffuse
   bleeding from an infected operative site   T
C. Hypotension is the earliest sign of hypovolaemia   F
D. The risk of deep venous thrombosis and pulmonary embolism
   is increased with malignancy   T
E. Acute tubular necrosis due to inadequate renal perfusion is
   irreversible   F

Q 5. Following major abdominal surgery

A. Epidural anaesthesia often masks the clinical signs of post-
   operative secondary haemorrhage   F
B. Insertion of a nasogastric tube prevents intestinal ileus   F
C. Swinging pyrexia and diarrhoea are characteristic clinical
   features of a pelvic abscess   T
D. Open drainage reduces the risk of septic complications   F
E. Subcutaneous heparin administration reduces the incidence
   of deep venous thrombosis   T

Q 6. Postoperative pyrexia may occur secondary to

A. Subphrenic abscess   T
B. Deep venous thrombosis   T
C. Urinary tract infection   T
D. Atelectasis   T
E. Blood transfusion   T

Q 7. The following are well-recognised specific postoperative complications

A. Renal failure in jaundiced patients   T
B. Deep venous thrombosis after varicose vein surgery   F
C. Hyperglycaemia, high lactate levels and a prolonged
   prothrombin time following liver resection for colorectal
   metastases   T
D. Positive Chvostek's sign after thyroid lobectomy   T
E. Urinary incontinence following inguinal hernia repair   F

Postoperative Management

Questions

Nutritional Support

Questions

Q 1. Parameters used to assess nutritional status include:

- A. Serum albumin   T
- B. Triceps skin-fold thickness   T
- C. White cell count   T
- D. Handgrip strength   T
- E. Prothrombin time   F

Q 2. Severe malnutrition is indicated by

- A. >10% recent weight loss   F
- B. Serum albumin <30 g/l   T
- C. Peripheral oedema   T
- D. Koilonychia   P
- E. Gynaecomastia   F

Q 3. Enteral nutrition

- A. Increases the incidence of bacterial translocation   F
- B. Maintains the gut mucosal barrier function   T
- C. May be safely administered immediately after abdominal surgery   F
- D. Should be considered the first choice of feeding for severe head injury patients   T
- E. Is associated with increased risk of infective complications compared to TPN-fed patients   F

Q 4. Daily nutritional requirements for a 70 kg man are:

- A. 35–40 kCal/kg/day   T
- B. 1–2 g nitrogen/day   F
- C. 15 g protein/day   F
- D. 70 mmol K$^+$/day   T
- E. 2500 ml water/day   T

Q 5. TPN

A. Most commonly is administered via large central veins   T

B. Is indicated in approx 25% of patients in hospital requiring F
nutritional support

C. Is indicated for all patients with paralytic ileus   F

D. Should be administered using an infusion pump   T

E. May induce hepatocyte dysfunction   T

Q 1. Features of the systemic inflammatory response syndrome (SIRS) include

  A. Temp >38.4°C
  B. Temp <35.6°C
  C. WCC <4 cells/ml
  D. Respiratory rate >20/min
  E. $PaCO_2$ >32 mmHg

Q 2. Factors which prevent overgrowth of pathogenic bacteria in the gastrointestinal tract include

  A. Small intestinal stasis
  B. Secretion of IgE
  C. Mucus production
  D. Antibiotics
  E. Blind loops

Q 3. Factors predisposing to nosocomial pneumonia include

  A. Oropharyngeal colonisation due to increased mouth breathing
  B. Routine use of H_2 antagonists
  C. Use of a nasogastric tube
  D. Endotracheal intubation
  E. Impaired gag reflex

Q 4. Systemic endotoxin may trigger the release of

  A. Pro-inflammatory cytokines
  B. Anti-inflammatory cytokines
  C. Complement
  D. Platelet activating factor (PAF)
  E. Endotoxin antibodies

Q 5. Factors predisposing to wound infection include

A. Inadequate haemostasis
B. Prolonged operation
C. Diabetes
D. Obstructive jaundice
E. Malnutrition

Q 6. Features of Adult Respiratory Distress Syndrome (ARDS) include

A. Increased lung compliance
B. Hypoxaemia associated with decreasing inspired oxygen concentration
C. Pulmonary infiltrates on a chest X-ray
D. Encephalopathy
E. Dyspnoea or tachypnoea

Q 7. Regarding antibiotics

A. Penicillins act by disrupting the peptidoglycan of the bacterial cell wall
B. Ampicillin is effective against pseudomonas infections
C. Cephalosporans are usually prescribed as a monotherapy
D. Vancomycin is the treatment of choice for MRSA
E. Aminoglycosides may cause nephrotoxicity

Q 8. Indications to isolate patients infected with HIV, HBV or HCV include those with

A. Bleeding oesophageal varices
B. Profuse diarrhoea
C. Urinary tract infections
D. Diabetes
E. Surgical drains

Q 1. **Injection of 1% lignocaine with 1 in 200,000 adrenaline is a useful form of anaesthesia for**

    A. Reducing a Smith's fracture
    B. Performing a Zadek's procedure
    C. Repair of an indirect inguinal hernia
    D. Central line insertion
    E. Insertion of a Seton suture

Q 2. **Diathermy**

    A. Produces coagulation by oscillation of tissue ions
    B. In bipolar form is useful at circumcision
    C. In monopolar form is useful to obtain haemostasis in grade IV liver injuries
    D. May cause burns at sites distant from the point of contact
    E. In NdYAG form is used to destroy lesions in the gastrointestinal tract

Q 3. **Wound healing**

    A. Is characterised by increased vascular permeability
    B. Is associated with release of growth factors and cytokines by leukocytes and macrophages
    C. Is characterised by wound contracture due to shortening of myofibrils
    D. Is retarded by vitamin A deficiency
    E. Is improved by nutrients

Q 4. **The following factors may adversely affect the healing of wounds**

    A. Exposure to ultraviolet light
    B. Obstructive jaundice
    C. Advanced neoplasia

D. Exposure to ionising radiation
E. Infection

Q 5. Wound infection rates

A. Are approximately 10% in clean wounds
B. Can be reduced by shaving the operative site 24 h prior to surgery
C. Can be reduced by minimizing the prehospital stay
D. Can be reduced by application of chlorhexidine or iodine preparations in theatre to the operative site
E. Are increased in patients with zinc deficiency

Q 6. Burn injuries

A. Involving 20% of body surface area can be managed by daily dressings by a district nurse
B. Involving the thorax may require escarotomy
C. Of partial thickness are often painless, but needle pricks can usually be felt
D. Requires fluid replacement of 2–4 ml/kg per percent body surface burn within the first 24 h
E. To the head and neck have the lowest mortality rates

Q 7. The general effects of burn injury are

A. Increased metabolic rate
B. Impaired immune function
C. Hypernatraemia
D. Hypoalbuminaemia
E. Impairment of gut barrier function

Q 8. Contemporary management of burn injuries includes

A. Early enteral feeding
B. Administration of broad-spectrum antibiotics to prevent colonisation of the burn site prior to skin grafting
C. Meshing of split-skin grafts to allow up to six times the potential coverage of the graft
D. Application of occlusive, nonabsorptive dressings which should be changed on a daily basis
E. Early release of contractures to allow early mobilisation and to obtain the best functional and aesthetic result

Trauma: General Principles of Management

Questions

Q 1. **When a casualty has severe facial injuries**

    A. An immediate danger to life is blood loss   F

    B. Transport to the casualty department should be in the supine   F
position

    C. Airway obstruction can occur due to inhaled blood   T

    D. Surgical cricothyroidotomy may be required due to   T
oedema

    E. Cervical spine injury should be considered after securing a   I
definitive airway

Q 2. **In the early assessment and resuscitation of a trauma
patient**

    A. Application of a tourniquet to control obvious external   F
blood loss from a limb is essential to minimise hypovolaemic
shock

    B. Airway patency ensures adequate ventilation   F

    C. A urinary catheter should be inserted if the patient is   F
unconscious

    D. A normal lateral cervical spine X-ray excludes a cervical spine   F
injury

    E. Nasotracheal intubation should be undertaken in the apnoeic   F
patient

Q 3. **In compensated hypovolaemia due to haemorrhage**

    A. There is no significant reduction of systemic blood   T
pressure

    B. The vital organs are inadequately perfused   F

    C. There will be associated bradycardia   F

    D. The patient may feel thirsty   T

    E. 1000 ml of blood may have been lost from the intravascular   T
compartment

Q 4. **Severe head injury may be associated with**

A. Raised systemic arterial blood pressure
B. No evidence of damage on CT scan
C. Secondary injury due to tissue hypoxia
D. Retention of carbon dioxide
E. A Glasgow Coma Score of 10

Q 5. **Indications for emergency thoracotomy include**

A. Patients with penetrating precordial injuries who are in EMD
B. Immediate evacuation of 750 ml blood on insertion of a chest drain
C. Continued blood loss from a chest drain of 200 ml/h for >3 h
D. A haemodynamically stable patient with a wide mediastinum on chest X-ray
E. A patient with hypoxia and a flail chest segment

Q 6. **Definite indications for emergency laparotomy are**

A. Stab wounds to the back with evidence of injury to the renal parenchyma
B. Gunshot wound to the abdomen
C. Stab wound to periumbilical region with protrusion of bowel
D. Haemodynamically stable patient with a liver laceration and free intra-abdominal fluid on CT scan
E. Injured diaphragm

Q 7. **Diagnostic peritoneal lavage (DPL)**

A. Is less sensitive than a CT scan for intraperitoneal bleeding
B. Is positive if the red cell count is >10,000 RBCs/mm^3
C. Is positive if the white cell count is >1000 WBCs/mm^3
D. Should be performed in a haemodynamically unstable patient with peritonism
E. Is positive if the aspirate contains bowel contents

Q 8. Liver injuries

A. Are predominantly due to blunt trauma in the UK
B. Due to deceleration forces, as in road traffic accidents, commonly cause lacerations between the anterior and posterior sectors of the right lobe of the liver
C. May result in hyperpyrexia
D. Frequently necessitate anatomical resection of the involved liver lobe
E. Can be managed by packing gauzes into hepatic lacerations and transferring the patient to a specialist liver unit for definitive surgical treatment

Q 9. In the management of burn injuries

A. Patients should receive 35% oxygen via a face mask if inhalation injury is suspected
B. 2–4 ml crystalloid per kilogram body weight per percent body surface burn is required in the first 24 h to maintain an adequate circulating blood volume
C. One half of the estimated fluid requirement for the first 24 h should be administered over the first 4 h
D. Prophylactic antibiotics are indicated in the early postburn period
E. Acid burns are generally more serious than alkali burns

Q 10. The metabolic response to injury includes

A. Increased ADH secretion
B. Elevation of serum growth hormone
C. Increased ACTH secretion from the hypothalamus
D. Transient hypoglycaemia in the early stage after injury
E. Increased urinary resorption of potassium

Q 1.   Cardiac output

    A. Is a function of stroke volume and mean arterial pressure   F
    B. Is regulated by the autonomic nervous system   T
    C. Is regulated by chemoreceptors   TF
    D. Can be measured by a thermodilutional technique   T
    E. Can increase to 40 L/min with exercise   T

Q 2.   Cardiac tamponade

    A. Is exacerbated by restrictive pulmonary disease   F
    B. May result from penetrating cardiac wounds   T
    C. Results in a low CVP   F
    D. Is associated with pulsus paradoxus   T
    E. Requires open surgical evacuation of blood and clot   F

Q 3.   The Adult Respiratory Distress Syndrome (ARDS)

    A. May occur following massive blood transfusion   T
    B. Is characterised by the development of radiological signs prior to clinical deterioration   F
    C. Is associated with the systemic inflammatory response syndrome (SIRS)   T
    D. Is associated with increased lung compliance   F
    E. Often requires respiratory support using artificial ventilation with positive end-expiratory pressure (PEEP)   T

Q 4.   Artificial ventilation

    A. Is indicated for type III respiratory failure
    B. Is best achieved with relatively low tidal volumes at a relatively fast rate
    C. For a short duration will be easier to be weaned from than that continued for a more prolonged period
    D. Necessitates paralysis of the patient
    E. May reduce venous return if PEEP is used

Q 5. **The Systemic Inflammatory Response Syndrome (SIRS)**

   A. Implies a focus of sepsis which must be localised and treated
   B. Rarely leads to end organ failure
   C. Stimulates fixed tissue macrophages to secrete cytokines
   D. May be associated with gut barrier dysfunction
   E. May be associated with a compensatory anti-inflammatory response

Q 6. **Acute renal failure**

   A. May cause a metabolic acidosis
   B. Is diagnosed when the urinary output falls below 800 ml in 24 h
   C. In critically ill patients should be treated by haemodialysis
   D. Is associated with hypokalaemia
   E. May be minimised by treating with a Dopamine infusion at 0.5–3 mg/kg/h

Q 7. **Acute liver failure may be associated with**

   A. Reduced systolic blood pressure
   B. Hyperglycaemia
   C. Hypernatraemia
   D. An increased prothrombin time
   E. Encephalopathy

Q 1. **Associations have been identified between the following carcinogens and cancer**

- **A.** Aflatoxin and pancreatic cancer   F
- **B.** Beta-carotene and stomach cancer   F
- **C.** Epstein-Barr virus and nasopharyngeal cancer   T
- **D.** Liver cirrhosis due to hepatitis C and hepatocellular carcinoma   T
- **E.** Human papilloma virus and endometrial cancer   F

Q 2. **With regard to a cancer screening test**

- **A.** The sensitivity of the test defines the proportion of those with cancer in whom a positive test has been recorded   T
- **B.** The specificity is the reciprocal of the false negative rate   F
- **C.** The specificity is the proportion of all those without cancer who are correctly classified as negative by the screening test   T
- **D.** Sensitivity and specificity are inversely related   F
- **E.** The positive predictive value represents the proportion of those with a positive test who are subsequently proven to have cancer   T

Q 3. **The following tumour markers are associated with specific tumours**

- **A.** Calcitonin and anaplastic thyroid cancer   F
- **B.** HCG and testicular teratoma   T
- **C.** Antidiuretic hormone and bronchogenic carcinoma   T
- **D.** Alpha-feto protein and liver metastases   F
- **E.** Carcinoembryonic antigen and rectal carcinoma   T

Q 4. **The following statements apply to the treatment of cancer**

- **A.** Brachytherapy involves the use of liquid nitrogen in the local treatment of malignant disease   F

B. Hyperbaric oxygen has been used as a radiosensitiser in radiation therapy   T

C. Photodynamic therapy can be used in the treatment of brain tumours   f

D. Neoadjuvant therapy is the application of new therapeutic strategies   f

E. Systemic chemotherapeutic agents may fail to cross the blood-brain barrier   T

Q 5. **The following are characteristic features of malignant tumours**

A. Pleomorphism   T

B. Anaplasia   T

C. Metaplasia   F

D. Reactive hyperplasia in local lymph nodes   f

E. Ulceration   T

Q 6. **Concerning specific neoplasms**

A. Small cell anaplastic tumours of the lung can secrete a variety of hormones   T

B. Hypernephroma may cause IVC obstruction secondary to progressive tumour growth from the renal vein   T

C. Gastric cancer may metastasise to the ovaries   T

D. Carcinoma of the caecum and ascending colon frequently presents with intestinal obstruction   F

E. Carcinoma of the tail of the pancreas can usually be resected by a distal pancreatectomy   T

Q 7. **These tumours secrete the following tumour markers**

A. Colorectal carcinoma – carcinoembryonic antigen (CEA)   T

B. Prostatic carcinoma – prostate specific antigen (PSA)   T

C. Cholangiocarcinoma – alpha-feto protein (AFP)   F

D. Testicular seminoma – human chorionic gonadotrophin (HCG)   T

E. Ovarian carcinoma – CA 125   T

Q 8. **The following conditions are premalignant**

A. Familial adenomatous polyposis   T

B. Barretts oesophagus   T

C. Keratoacanthoma   F

D. Gastric fundic gland polyps   F

E. Plummer-Vinson syndrome   F

Q 1. **Concerning consent for surgery**

   A. In British Law, anyone over the age of 16 years is regarded as potentially able to give consent   F

   B. If a patient is mentally incapable of giving consent (e.g. due to senile dementia), consent can be given by a first degree relative   F

   C. If a patient is physically incapable of giving consent (e.g. an unconscious patient), consent can be given by a first degree relative   F

   D. Consent for an operation generally applies to all aspects and procedures related to the operation   T

   E. If a parent refuses essential treatment for a child, the doctor must adhere to this and cannot in any way undertake treatment of the child   F

Q 1. **The following are examples of inflammatory mediators**

- **A.** Platelet-Derived Growth Factor (PDGF)
- **B.** Tumour Necrosis Factor (TNF)
- **C.** Interleukin 6
- **D.** Erythropoietin
- **E.** Leucotriene B_4

Q 2. **Which of the following statements are true**

- **A.** Pulse oximeters are not accurate in patients with a haemoglobin less than 5 g/dL
- **B.** Approximately 60% of the body's excess iron is stored in the bone marrow
- **C.** Red blood cells for transfusion can be stored for up to 90 days at 4°C
- **D.** Disseminated intravascular coagulation (DIC) is characterized by an increase in the platelet count and an increase in fibrin degradation products
- **E.** Disseminated intravascular coagulation (DIC) results in an increased clotting tendency and an increased risk of venous thrombosis

Q 3. **The following statements are true**

- **A.** Splenectomy results in a decreased platelet count
- **B.** Splenectomy results in an increased incidence of infection
- **C.** Idiopathic thrombocytopaenic purpura is a common indication for splenectomy
- **D.** Trauma to the spleen is an absolute indication for splenectomy
- **E.** Implantation of diced pieces of splenic tissue into the omentum after splenectomy results in immunologically functioning splenic tissue

Alimentary System — Questions

Q 1. The transpyloric plane

A. Is an imaginary line running between the tips of the seventh costal cartilages

B. Identifies the level at which the superior mesenteric vein joins the splenic vein to form the portal vein

C. Defines the level of the neck of the pancreas

D. Corresponds to the level of L3 posteriorly

E. Defines the level of entry of the cystic duct into the common bile duct

Q 2. Oesophageal pH monitoring

A. Should be performed at the level of the gastro-oesophageal junction

B. Is indicated in patients with gastro-oesophageal reflux disease

C. Which reveals a pH <4 for more than 4% of a 24 h period is diagnostic for pathological reflux

D. Should be performed following anti-reflux surgery

E. Is helpful to diagnose Zollinger-Ellison Syndrome

Q 3. An ileostomy

A. Typically produces 1500–2000 ml small intestinal content per day

B. May be associated with vitamin B12 deficiency

C. Is often fashioned following panproctocolectomy perfomed for inflammatory bowel disease

D. Should preferably be designed as a spout as this promotes the bowel contents to become more formed in nature

E. Is associated with an increased incidence of gallstones and renal calculi

Q 4. Regarding abdominal stomas

A. A gastrostomy may be used as an alternative to an NG tube following laparotomy for severe necrotising pancreatitis

B. A PEG tube is often used to enterally feed a patient with malignant oesophageal obstruction

C. The management of a temporary proximal defunctioning colostomy is equivalent to the management of an end colostomy using the descending colon

D. A defunctioning loop ileostomy reduces the anastomotic leak rate following a low anterior resection

E. Enteral feeding via a jejunostomy reduces the incidence of postoperative nosocomial infections following major abdominal surgery

Q 5. Concerning trauma assessment and resuscitation

A. The primary survey involves assessment of gastrointestinal and urological injuries

B. Immediate laparotomy is indicated for a patient with localised peritonism in the left upper quadrant following blunt abdominal trauma

C. A plain abdominal X-ray is mandatory to exclude a ruptured hollow viscus following blunt abdominal trauma

D. CT scanning is essential for patients with generalised abdominal pain and persistent hypotension to define the site of an intra-abdominal injury

E. Omentum protruding through an abdominal stab wound is an absolute indication for laparotomy

Q 6. Concerning liver trauma

A. The liver is the most frequently injured solid intra-abdominal organ following blunt trauma

B. Penetrating liver injuries require exploratory laparotomy

C. Liver lacerations associated with haemodynamic instability and coagulopathy should be managed by inserting packs into the lacerations to control haemorrhage

D. The Pringle manoeuvre can be used for up to 60 minutes to control haemorrhage from the liver

E. Sepsis following liver trauma is a significant cause of late mortality in multiply injured patients

Q 7. Common causes of acute abdominal pain are

- **(A.)** Diverticulitis   T
- **B.** Meckels diverticulum   F
- **(C.)** Cholecystitis   T
- **(D.)** Appendicitis   T
- **E.** Mesenteric ischaemia   T

Q 8. With regard to an appendix mass

- **A.** Surgery is indicated if ultrasonography detects a collection of   F
  pus within the inflammatory mass
- **(B.)** Patients should generally be administered intravenous   T
  antibiotics and managed conservatively
- **(C.)** After resolution of appendix mass in an elderly patient,   T
  barium enema or colonoscopy should be used to exclude
  underlying caecal carcinoma
- **(D.)** The differential diagnosis includes Crohns disease and a   T
  caecal tumour
- **E.** Delayed appendicectomy is mandatory   F

Q 9. Useful investigations in patients with an acute abdomen include

- **(A.)** Laparoscopy   F
- **B.** Peritoneal lavage   F
- **(C.)** Ultrasound   T
- **D.** Abdominal X-ray to diagnose gallstones   F
- **(E.)** Serum amylase   T

Q 10. Concerning acute cholecystitis

- **A.** May be associated with a bradycardia   F
- **(B.)** May be associated with a positive Murphy's sign   T
- **C.** Typically presents with periumbilical pain localising to the   F
  right hypochondrium
- **(D.)** May be treated by laparoscopic cholecystectomy within 72 h   F
  of admission
- **(E.)** In elderly unfit patients, insertion of a radiologically-guided   T
  percutaneous drain into the gallbladder may allow symptoms
  to settle

Q 11. Concerning acute pancreatitis

- **A.** No aetiological factor may be identified in up to 20% of patients
- **B.** May be associated with a normal amylase concentration
- **C.** May be secondary to pancreatic carcinoma
- **D.** Evidence of pancreatic necrosis on CT scan is an indication for necrosectomy
- **E.** If gallstones are implicated, laparoscopic cholecystectomy should be performed 3–6 months after complete resolution of inflammation

Q 12. Small bowel obstruction

- **A.** Is most often due to an external hernia
- **B.** May result in a metabolic alkalosis or a metabolic acidosis
- **C.** May result in hyperkalaemia
- **D.** May settle with conservative treatment
- **E.** Due to gallstone ileus will often be associated with gas in the biliary tree

Q 13. Obstructive jaundice

- **A.** May be due to portal lymphadenopathy
- **B.** Is associated with an increased risk of postoperative septic complications and renal dysfunction
- **C.** Due to a periampullary tumour may be associated with silvery stools
- **D.** Secondary to a Klatskin tumour is usually treated by segmental liver resection and excision of the involved extrahepatic biliary tree
- **E.** Which develops following laparoscopic cholecystectomy should be investigated by cholangiography

Q 14. Concerning gallstones

- **A.** Recurrent obstruction and infection in the biliary tree due to gallstones may result in primary biliary cirrhosis
- **B.** Biliary obstruction of the common hepatic duct by gallstones may produce a mucocele of the gallbladder
- **C.** Passage of a gallstone through the Sphincter of Oddi may result in a gallstone ileus

D. A gallstone impacted at Hartman's pouch will usually cause obstructive jaundice

E. Gallstones causing obstructive jaundice can be demonstrated by intravenous cholangiography

Q 15. Aetiological factors associated with peptic ulceration include

A. Head injury
B. *Helicobacter pylori* infection
C. Gastrinoma
D. Bile reflux
E. High intragastric pH

Q 16. Current treatment for peptic ulceration includes

A. Antibiotics
B. H^+K^+ ATPase inhibition
C. Prostaglandin antagonists
D. H_2 receptor antagonists
E. Vagotomy and gastrojejunostomy

Q 17. Achalasia

A. Classically results in a dilated sigmoid-shaped oesophagus as seen on barium swallow
B. Characteristically is associated with a lower oesophageal sphincter pressure of >40 mmHg
C. Is associated with an increased risk of oesophageal malignancy
D. Can be treated by injection of Botulinum toxin
E. Is due to degeneration of the myenteric plexus

Q 18. Concerning inguinal hernias

A. Indirect are more common than direct
B. If direct, they exit the peritoneal cavity between the inguinal ligament, inferior epigastric vessels and the lateral border of the rectus abdominus muscle.
C. If direct, is usually due to degenerative factors
D. If indirect, enters the deep inguinal ring medial to the inferior epigastric vessels

E. Indirect are more likely to develop complications, such as strangulation or obstruction

Q 19. Femoral hernias

A. Are the commonest type of groin hernia in females
B. Rarely develop complications
C. Occur more commonly in women than men
D. Are repaired by suturing Cooper's ligament to the inguinal ligament
E. Project through the femoral canal which is lateral to the femoral vein

Q 20. Oesophageal carcinoma

A. Commonly presents with bleeding
B. Is usually an adenocarcinoma
C. May arise in a segment of Barrett's metaplasia
D. Involving the lower third of the oesophagus may spread to the coeliac trunk lymph nodes
E. May be palliated by insertion of an expandable metal stent

Q 21. Aetiological factors for gastric cancer include

A. High socio-economic class
B. Previous partial gastrectomy
C. Pernicious anaemia
D. Blood group O
E. Smoking

Q 22. Recognised associations with gastric carcinoma include

A. Linitis plastica
B. Troisier's sign
C. Gastric volvulus
D. Krukenberg's tumours
E. Migratory thrombophlebitis

Q 23. Pancreatic carcinoma

A. Commonly presents with an epigastric mass
B. Is associated with acanthosis nigricans

C. Is resectable in approximately 50% of cases

D. May be diagnosed by a double duct sign at ERCP

E. Is associated with a 5-year survival of 50–60% following Whipple pancreaticoduodenectomy

Q 24. Colorectal cancer

A. Is the commonest cause of male cancer deaths in the Western world

B. Classified as Duke's stage B has spread through the bowel wall

C. With liver metastases is incurable

D. Has a family history in 25% of cases

E. Is associated with a 5-year survival of 90% if classified as Duke's stage A

Q 1. Factors which lead to an increase in blood viscosity include

(A.) Polycythaemia
B. Hypofibrinogenaemia
(C.) Leukaemia
D. Cryoglobinaemia
(E.) Dehydration

Q 2. Principle causes of acute ischaemia include

A. Diabetes
(B.) Embolism
(C.) Thrombosis
D. Atheroma
(E.) Arteritis

Q 3. Chronic arterial atheromatous disease typically affects the following arteries

(A.) Cerebral
B. Radial
(C.) Renal
(D.) Aorta
(E.) Iliac

Q 4. Concerning the ankle/brachial pressure index

(A.) It is measured using a sphygmomanometer cuff and stethoscope
(B.) The pressure at the ankle should be the same or higher than the brachial pressure
C. An index of approximately 0.7 indicates severe ischaemia
D. The pressure at the ankle in diabetics is usually higher than the arm

E. All patients with proven occlusive disease will have abnormal resting pressures

Q 5. The following statements concerning aneurysms are true

A. An aortic aneurysm >6 cm should be treated
B. A dissecting aneurysm occurs due to destruction of the vessel intima
C. A true aneurysm is covered by all 3 layers of the vessel wall
D. An aortic aneurysm usually occurs above the level of the renal arteries
E. A patient with an aortic aneurysm who is deemed unfit for surgical repair should undergo attempted surgical repair if rupture occurs

Q 6. The following statements concerning arterial surgery are true

A. Transluminal angioplasty is most successful in the popliteal arteries
B. Transluminal angioplasty is successful in asymmetrical stenoses
C. Transluminal angioplasty is not of value in calcified stenoses
D. Indications for sympathectomy include palmar and pedal hyperhidrosis and ischaemic cutaneous ulceration
E. Endarterectomy is the procedure of choice at the carotid bifurcation

Q 7. The following statements concerning venous disease are true

A. Primary or familial varicose veins occur in approximately 40% of patients
B. Arterial disease accounts for approximately 40% of leg ulcers
C. Chronic venous ulceration is usually treated by calf perforator ligation
D. Chronic ulceration should be treated by a trial of antibiotics (eg flucloxacillin)
E. Chronic ulcers should be dressed with de sloughing agents

Endocrine Surgery   Questions

Q 1. **Embryological abnormalities of development of the thyroid gland include**

- **A.** Reidel's lobe
- **B.** Thyroglossal cyst
- **C.** Retrosternal goitre
- **D.** Lobar agenesis
- **E.** Foramen caecum

Q 2. **Which of the following statements regarding normal thyroid physiology is/are true**

- **A.** 98% of absorbed iodide is taken up by the thyroid gland
- **B.** Approximately 80 mg of free thyroxine is formed per day
- **C.** The majority of T4 in the tissues is formed by the conversion of T3 to T4
- **D.** Thyroid secretion is controlled by TSH, which is released from the posterior pituitary gland
- **E.** The biological half-life of thyroxine is 6 h

Q 3. **The main effects of thyroxine are**

- **A.** Regulation of body basal metabolic rate
- **B.** Increase in tissue oxygen consumption
- **C.** Regulation of gastrointestinal hormone secretion
- **D.** Influence on growth and maturation
- **E.** Increase absorption of carbohydrate from the intestine

Q 4. **Symptoms suggestive of thyroid malignancy include**

- **A.** Rapid onset of a painful neck swelling
- **B.** Dysphagia
- **C.** Development of hoarseness
- **D.** Weight gain
- **E.** Cervical lymphadenopathy

Q 5. Symptoms of hyperthyroidism include

   A. Bradycardia
   B. Atrial fibrillation
   C. Anorexia
   D. Weight gain
   E. Tremor

Q 6. Treatment of thyrotoxicosis may include

   A. Carbamazepine
   B. Radioiodine administration
   C. Propylthiouracil
   D. Thyroid lobectomy
   E. Thyroxine

Q 7. Postoperative complications associated with thyroidectomy include

   A. Hypercalcaemia
   B. Reactionary haemorrhage
   C. Hypothyroidism
   D. External laryngeal nerve palsy
   E. Pituitary adenoma formation

Q 8. Causes of diffuse non-toxic goitre include:

   A. Pregnancy
   B. Iodine deficiency
   C. Laryngitis
   D. Myxoedema
   E. Polycystic disease

Q 9. Indications for surgery in patients with multinodular goitre include

   A. Hypothyroidism
   B. Increase in size of a dominant nodule
   C. Hypercalcaemia
   D. Retrosternal extension
   E. Cosmetic appearance

Q 10. Indicate whether the following statements are true or false

    A. 70% of solitary thyroid nodules are malignant

    B. Thyroid cysts can be treated by aspiration only

    C. The cytology of follicular adenoma and follicular carcinoma is identical

    D. Thyroid lobectomy is an adequate oncological procedure for papillary thyroid carcinoma

    E. Hypernephroma is responsible for most cases of secondary tumour deposits in the thyroid

Q 11. With regard to thyroid malignancy

    A. Thyroid lymphoma is treated primarily by surgical excision

    B. Medullary carcinoma may be associated with hyperparathyroidism

    C. Patients with a treated papillary carcinoma can expect a normal life expectancy

    D. Follicular carcinoma arises most commonly in middle-aged males

    E. Invasive follicular carcinoma may metastasise to bone

Q 12. Indicate whether the following statements are true or false

    A. The adrenal cortex produces noradrenaline and adrenaline

    B. Cortisol and corticosterone are powerful mineralocorticoids produced by the zona glomerulosa

    C. Catecholamine release is stimulated by the sympathetic nervous system

    D. Noradrenaline causes peripheral vasoconstriction

    E. Glucocorticoids are controlled primarily by secretion of adrenocorticotrophic hormone (ACTH)

Q 13. Cushing's disease is associated with

    A. Hypotension

    B. Pituitary tumour

    C. Skin pigmentation

    D. Moon face and buffalo hump

    E. Excessive diuresis

Q 14. Primary hyperaldosteronism

- **(A.)** Is most commonly due to an adrenal adenoma
- **B.** Is associated with high plasma renin levels
- **(C.)** May present with hypertension
- **(D.)** May be treated initially by spironolactone
- **E.** May be complicated by hyperkalaemia

Q 15. Parathormone

- **(A.)** Is produced by chief cells and oxyphil cells of the parathyroid gland
- **B.** Reduces serum calcium
- **C.** Increases phosphate reabsorption in the kidney
- **(D.)** Is measured by radioimmunoassay
- **(E.)** Secretion is inhibited by prolonged hypomagnesaemia

Q 16. Insulinoma

- **(A.)** Are usually benign tumours of the pancreas
- **(B.)** Often present with Whipple's triad
- **(C.)** May not be identified and localised prior to surgical exploration
- **(D.)** Can be treated by enucleation
- **E.** May be part of the Zollinger-Ellison syndrome

Q 17. Carcinoid tumours

- **A.** Most commonly arise in the pancreas
- **B.** Are usually symptomatic because of endocrine secretion at the time of presentation
- **C.** Metastasise to the liver in >50% of patients
- **(D.)** Produce excess serotonin
- **(E.)** Should be treated by resection of the primary tumour

Q 1. **With regard to investigation of symptomatic breast disease**

    A. Mammography is more accurate in elderly females compared to younger females

    B. Microcalcification is pathognomonic of breast malignancy

    C. Fine needle aspiration cytology (FNAC) is only useful for diagnosis of palpable breast lumps

    D. Triple assessment should achieve results with a sensitivity and specificity of >95%

    E. Excisional breast biopsy should be performed using a radial incision

Q 2. **Nipple discharge**

    A. Which is blood-stained is always due to breast cancer

    B. May be physiological

    C. May be bilateral in patients with prolactinaemia

    D. Is common in patients with Mondor's disease

    E. Due to an intraductal papilloma may require a microdochectomy

Q 3. **Causes of nipple retraction/inversion are**

    A. Mammary duct ectasia

    B. Paget's disease

    C. Congenital

    D. Trauma

    E. Fibrocystic disease

Q 4. **Breast pain**

    A. Is a presenting feature in 10% of patients with breast malignancy

    B. Can be treated with gamma-Linolenic acid with minimal side effects

C. May be due to Tietz's syndrome
D. Is effectively relieved by diuretics
E. If incapacitating may necessitate partial mastectomy of the affected region

Q 5. Mammary duct ectasia

A. Means that the ducts are dilated with mucus
B. Is premalignant
C. Usually presents with nipple retraction
D. Is treated by microdochectomy
E. Is characteristically associated with bacterial infection

Q 6. Pathophysiological changes associated with mammary dysplasia include

A. Metaplasia
B. Sclerosing adenosis
C. Epitheliosis
D. Cyst formation
E. Necrosis

Q 7. Gynaecomastia is associated with

A. Acute liver failure
B. Testicular cancer
C. Congenital testicular absence
D. Spironolactone
E. Puberty

Q 8. The following statements apply to benign breast disorders

A. Mammography should be performed in all patients with a palpable lump
B. Mammography can differentiate between fat necrosis and breast carcinoma
C. All fibroadenomas should be removed irrespective of size
D. Phylloides tumours can metastasise
E. Breast cysts are best diagnosed on ultrasound rather than mammography

Q 9. With regard to breast carcinoma

    A. Delayed menarche is a known risk factor

    B. Ductal carcinoma is more commonly multifocal than lobular carcinoma

    C. The most important prognostic factor is the size of the tumour

    D. Axillary clearance combined with axillary radiotherapy significantly reduces the likelihood of regional lymph node recurrence

    E. Oestrogen-receptor negative tumours respond better to Tamoxifen treatment than oestrogen-receptor positive tumours

Q 10. In the clinical staging of a breast cancer by the TNM classification, a staging of T2 N2 M1 indicates that

    A. The tumour is greater than 5 cm in diameter

    B. The tumour is fixed to the chest wall

    C. The ipsilateral internal mammary lymph nodes are involved

    D. Distant metastases are present

    E. Paget's disease is a possible diagnosis

Questions

Thoracic Surgery   Questions

Q 1. **Concerning pneumothorax**

  A. It is always due to blunt or penetrating chest trauma
  B. It should always be treated by intercostal tube drainage
  C. It can only occur if air enters a pleural space from the exterior or from the lung
  D. It should be treated by insertion of an intercostal tube drain in the mid-clavicular line, at the 2nd intercostal space
  E. When the pneumothorax is treated by chest tube drainage, the tube should be inserted beneath the rib above

Q 2. **Concerning infections of the chest and lungs**

  A. An empyema refers to a large collection of pus within one or more lobes of the lung
  B. An empyema may lead ultimately to fibrosis around the lung with restriction of expansion
  C. An empyema and bronchiectasis may be associated with finger clubbing
  D. Bronchiectasis most commonly affects the upper lobes of the lung
  E. Bronchiectasis is generally treated by postural drainage and antibiotics

Q 3. **Lung cancer**

  A. May be associated with venous engorgement of the face, arms and anterior chest wall
  B. May be associated with a Cushinoid appearance
  C. May be associated with Horner's syndrome if the lesion is close to the hilum
  D. Affects men more frequently than women with a ratio of 2:1
  E. Is most frequently an adenocarcinoma

Q 4. Concerning thoracic trauma

A. Aortic rupture should be suspected if there is widening of the upper mediastinum on a chest X-ray

B. Rib fracture alone is not associated with significant morbidity or mortality

C. The fracture of 3 or more ribs results in a flail chest

D. Approximately 85% of patients with a haemothorax require a thoracotomy

E. Rupture of the diaphragm may be diagnosed on chest X-ray

Q 1. Adenocarcinoma of the kidney

    A. Most commonly occurs in women
    B. Responds well to chemotherapy
    C. May present with a pathological fracture
    D. Arises in the glomeruli
    E. May be associated with a right sided varicocele

Q 2. Causes of hydronephrosis include

    A. PUJ obstruction
    B. Stone
    C. Tumour
    D. Stricture
    E. Paraphimosis

Q 3. Transitional cell carcinoma

    A. Classically presents with painless haematuria
    B. Does not respond to chemoradiotherapy
    C. Occurs more frequently in smokers
    D. Of the bladder should be treated by cystectomy and urinary diversion if the tumour has not invaded the muscle wall
    E. Is usually not associated with urinary infection

Q 4. Urinary retention

    A. May result in renal dysfunction
    B. Occurring in young females is usually not associated with any significant underlying pathology
    C. Is invariably associated with suprapubic pain
    D. Due to urethral stricture is best managed by suprapubic catheterisation
    E. May occur in patients with normal transurethral endoscopic findings

Q 5. Benign nodular hyperplasia of the prostate

A. Most commonly presents with hesitancy, poor stream and post micturitional dribbling

B. Is due to development of a large adenoma rather than diffuse prostatic hypertrophy

C. When treated by transurethral resection, results in sterility

D. May be treated non-surgically

E. Is usually due to a chronic viral infection

Q 6. Carcinoma of the prostate

A. Usually presents at an early stage

B. Is the second commonest cause of cancer deaths in males

C. Has a specific tumour marker

D. Frequently causes lytic bony metastases

E. May be treated by hormone manipulation

Q 7. Concerning testicular swellings

A. A hydatid of Morgagni is a small cystic remnant at the upper pole of the testis

B. A hydrocele usually has multiple septae

C. Needle drainage of a hydrocele usually provides long-term resolution

D. A varicocele is treated by excision of the peri-testicular pampiniform venous plexus

E. Orchitis and torsion can be reliably distinguished clinically

Q 8. Concerning testicular tumours

A. A solid swelling of the testis should be presumed malignant until proved otherwise

B. Teratoma occurs in a younger age group than seminoma

C. Serum alpha-feto protein and beta-human chorionic gonadotrophin concentrations are abnormal in 75% of cases of teratoma

D. Seminoma is not radiosensitive

E. Teratoma does not respond to chemotherapy

Q 1.   Basal cell carcinoma

    A. Should be treated primarily by radiotherapy
    B. May present as an ulcer or as a thickened plaque
    C. Is the commonest skin cancer
    D. Of the face occurs most commonly below the line between the angle of the mouth and the pinna
    E. Should be treated by surgical excision with a 5 mm clearance margin

Q 2.   Concerning cancers of the head and neck

    A. 90% are squamous carcinomas
    B. Carcinoma of the tongue tends to metastasise early
    C. Surgery and chemotherapy are the principal treatment modalities
    D. Mouth cancer is often associated with elevated levels of antibodies to Epstein-Barr virus
    E. The peak age incidence for melanoma is 60–65 years

Q 3.   The following are differential diagnoses of a midline neck swelling

    A. Submental lymph node
    B. Laryngocele
    C. Branchial cyst
    D. Cystic hygroma
    E. Dermoid cyst

Q 4.   A thyroglossal cyst

    A. Moves up on protrusion of the tongue
    B. Is treated by incision and drainage
    C. Classically occurs in the midline
    D. Is prone to infection
    E. Often contains cholesterol crystals

Q 5. A branchial cyst

A. May be confused with nodal metastasis
B. Is treated by aspiration
C. Is derived from ectoderm of the second branchial pouch
D. Is lined with squamous epithelium and contains cholesterol crystals
E. Classically occurs in the midline

Q 6. The following are true of salivary neoplasms

A. Approximately 10% of parotid gland tumours are malignant
B. A Wharthin's tumour is a benign lesion
C. Adenoid cystic carcinomas of the parotid are the commonest malignancy
D. Pleomorphic salivary adenomas are well encapsulated and thus are best treated by local excision
E. Open incisional biopsy is recommended for diagnosis of parotid tumours

Q 7. The following are well recognised complications after surgery to the head and neck

A. Gustatory sweating after superficial parotidectomy
B. Sialorrhoea (dribbling from the angle of the mouth) after excision of the submandibular gland
C. Exposure keratitis after parotid surgery
D. Horner's syndrome after total parotidectomy
E. Shoulder drop and weakness of the deltopectoral girdle after radical lymph node dissection of the neck

Q 1. **The Glasgow Coma Scale**

A. Measures 4 patient responses: eye opening, verbal response, motor response and pupillary reflexes
B. Defines coma as a response <8
C. Is used principally as a one off test to rapidly document the level of consciousness
D. If less than 6, represents an indication for exploratory burr-holes
E. May be used to diagnose an intracerebral haematoma

Q 2. **Increased intracranial pressure may typically be asssociated with**

A. Tachycardia
B. Hypotension
C. Apnoea
D. Transtentorial herniation
E. Foraminal herniation

Q 3. **Chronic subdural haematoma**

A. Is usually associated with a head injury
B. Is more likely to occur in chronic alcoholics
C. Is associated with fluctuating confusion and drowsiness
D. May mimic a stroke
E. Is usually associated with a skull fracture

Q 4. **In a multiply traumatised patient with a head injury**

A. An immediate skull X-ray is mandatory
B. The pupillary response is the most important physical sign in terms of assessment of the head injury
C. Intravenous dexamethasone infusion should be commenced immediately

    D. Restlessness, confusion and aggression indicate that the patient has a very severe head injury

    E. Management of the head injury takes priority over management of other injuries

Q 5. **The following statements are true**

    A. Cerebral abscess is usually due to haematogenous spread

    B. Approximately 50% of intracranial tumours are metastatic

    C. Meningiomas frequently metastasise

    D. In an acute head injury, a unilateral, fixed, dilated pupil is always caused by a haematoma

    E. An extradural haematoma is usually associated with rupture of the vertebral artery

Q 1. **Fracture healing is adversely affected in the following situations**

  A. Elderly patients
  B. Poor nutritional status
  C. The presence of a gap between the fracture ends
  D. Interposition of soft tissue between the fracture ends
  E. A slight degree of mobility between the fracture ends

Q 2. **The following statements concerning fracture healing are true**

  A. Delayed union refers to fracture healing which takes longer than normal
  B. Non-union refers to complete failure of a fracture to unite
  C. Mal-union refers to a fracture which unites but in a non-anatomical position
  D. Hypertrophic union refers to excessive callus formation which becomes ossified
  E. A pathological fracture refers to a fracture which occurs in bone weakened by pre-existing disease

Q 3. **Avascular necrosis is a well recognised complication of the following fractures**

  A. Neck of femur
  B. Shaft of femur
  C. Scaphoid
  D. Calcaneus
  E. Hamate

Q 4. **Concerning bone and joint infections**

  A. Acute osteomyelitis is usually due to Salmonella
  B. Acute osteomyelitis is characterized by local pain, generalised sweating, fever, malaise and anorexia

C. Acute septic arthritis is usually due to pseudomonas

D. Acute septic arthritis should be treated by urgent decompression and lavage of the joint plus intravenous antibiotics

E. Suspected acute septic arthritis should be investigated by aspiration of the joint fluid for culture

Q 1. Concerning oesophageal atresia and tracheo-oesophageal fistula (TOF)

A. The most frequent type is a proximal oesophageal atresia with a distal tracheo-oesophageal fistula
B. There is a high incidence of associated anomalies
C. It may be associated with maternal polyhydramnios
D. Treatment involves a right thoracotomy and anastomosis of the oesophagus
E. It affects 1 in 100 live births

Q 2. Gastro-oesophageal reflux

A. Is uncommon in infants
B. Usually resolves with simple measures
C. May present with respiratory symptoms
D. May present with upper GI bleeding
E. Very rarely requires surgical treatment

Q 3. The following statements are true

A. Pyloric atresia is treated by resection and anastomosis
B. Duodenal atresia is commonly associated with Downs syndrome
C. Meconium ileus occurs in approximately 50% of children with cystic fibrosis
D. Neonatal intestinal obstruction is characterised by bilious vomiting, abdominal distension and failure to pass meconium
E. Anorectal atresia is more common in boys than girls

Q 4. .The following statements are true

A. Infantile hypertrophic pyloric stenosis is the commonest cause of non-bilious vomiting in infants

B. In equivocal cases of infantile pyloric stenosis, where a pyloric tumour is not palpable, a barium meal is the investigation of choice

C. Pyloric stenosis should be treated by immediate/emergency laparotomy

D. Intussusception occurs most frequently in the 2–3 year age group

E. Ileo-ileal is the most frequent type of intussusception

Q 5. The following statements are true

A. In gastroschisis there is no peritoneal sac and eviscerated bowel is exposed to amniotic fluid during intrauterine life

B. Gastroschisis and exomphalos should be treated by primary fascial repair

C. Four types of biliary atresia are recognised

D. The best results for the Kasai operation for biliary atresia are achieved before age 6–8 weeks

E. Choledochal cyst should be treated by drainage into a loop of jejunum

Q 6. The following statements concerning scrotal and groin disorders in children are true

A. Inguinal hernia in a child is treated by herniorrhaphy

B. Hydrocele in a child is treated by the Jaboulay procedure

C. Testicular torsion is twice as common on the left side

D. Surgery for testicular torsion is an absolute surgical emergency

E. Undescended testes affects 4–5% of boys

Preoperative Management

Answers

A 1.   **A.** true   **B.** false   **C.** true   **D.** true   **E.** true

Mild to moderate systemic disturbance which does not limit normal activity is ASA 2.

ASA 3 refers to severe systemic disturbance which limits normal activity but is not incapacitating.

Fundamentals of Surgical Practice Chapter 1.

A 2.   **A.** true   **B.** true   **C.** false   **D.** true   **E.** false

A 3.   **A.** false   **B.** true   **C.** true   **D.** true   **E.** false

The WHO defines hypertension as a diastolic pressure of >95 mmHg.

Fundamentals of Surgical Practice Chapter 1.

A 4.   **A.** false   **B.** false   **C.** true   **D.** false   **E.** true

There is a risk of adrenal suppression (with Addisonian crisis) and cover with IV hydrocortisone (100 mg bd) should be used during the perioperative period.

The progesterone-only oral contraceptive pill has no documented risk during surgery but the combination estrogen-progesterone pill should be discontinued 6 weeks prior to elective surgery because of the risk of DVT, particularly in women who smoke.

Aspirin should be discontinued 2 weeks prior to elective surgery.

Antihypertensives should be continued up to the time of surgery.

Warfarin should be discontinued and heparin prophylaxis should be initiated.

Fundamentals of Surgical Practice Chapter 1.

A 5. **A.** false **B.** false **C.** false **D.** false **E.** true

An ECG should be performed on all patients with known cardiovascular disease but only routinely on asymptomatic patients >60 years.

A chest X-ray is one of the commonest preoperative investigations to be performed but it rarely detects unexpected pathology.

A biochemical screen rarely reveals unexpected pathology. Each surgical unit will have its own policy/protocol for these but, as a general principle, excessive preoperative investigation in healthy patients represents a waste of resources and should be discouraged.

Elevation of the GGT or Alk Phos may be due to the presence of bile duct stones and thus an operative cholangiogram will be indicated (if a cholangiogram has not previously been performed endoscopically (ERCP)).

Fundamentals of Surgical Practice Chapter 1.

A 6. **A.** true **B.** false **C.** true **D.** true **E.** false

Halving the dose of depot insulin on the day prior to surgery avoids hypoglycaemia on the day of surgery, due to the effects of long-acting insulin.

No insulin is given prior to surgery as hypoglycaemia is the major risk on the day of operation.

An intravenous infusion of 5% dextrose erected on the morning of surgery avoids hypoglycaemia on the day of operation.

Due to increased output of glucocorticoids, which have an anti-insulin effect, insulin requirements may increase after major surgery.

The majority of diabetic patients undergoing surgery have Non-Insulin Dependent Diabetes Mellitus (NIDDM or Type II diabetes).

Fundamentals of Surgical Practice Chapter 1.

A **7.** **A.** false **B.** true **C.** true **D.** false **E.** false

Enoxaparin is a low molecular weight heparin and is given only once daily (20 mg/day).

Non-significant thrombolism occurs in up to 30% of patients.

Electrical calf stimulators or pneumatic leg compressors contribute significantly to reduce the incidence of thromboembolism.

Although it is effective, Dextran 70 is currently too expensive to allow widespread usage.

Age >40 years is a significant risk factor for the development of deep vein thrombosis.

Fundamentals of Surgical Practice Chapter 1.

A 1. **A.** true **B.** true **C.** false **D.** true **E.** false

Sevoflurane and halothane are inhalational agents.

Fundamentals of Surgical Practice Chapter 2.

A 2. **A.** true **B.** false **C.** false **D.** false **E.** false

Only suxamethonium is a depolarising agent and acts by mimicking the action of acetylcholine. The others are non-depolarising agents and act by binding reversibly to cholinergic receptors, thus preventing acetylcholine from activating them.

Fundamentals of Surgical Practice Chapter 2.

A 3. **A.** false **B.** true **C.** false **D.** true **E.** false

Morphine is a naturally occurring alkaloid.

Papavertum contains a mixture of morphine, thebaine and papaverine.

Fentanyl has little effect on the cardiovascular system.

Fundamentals of Surgical Practice Chapter 2.

A 4. **A.** true **B.** false **C.** false **D.** false **E.** false

NaCl 0.9% contains 154 mmol of chloride per litre.

Glucose 5% does not contain any electrolytes.

Hartmann's contains 5 mmol of potassium per litre but does not contain any calories. Glucose 5% contains 188 kCal/L.

Fundamentals of Surgical Practice Chapter 2.

A 5.　**A.** true　**B.** true　**C.** false　**D.** false　**E.** false

Sympathetic blockade may cause a loss of vascular smooth muscle tone with consequent decrease in vascular resistance, fall in blood pressure, venous return and cardiac output.

Blockade of motor function may be very distressing for the patient.

Fundamentals of Surgical Practice Chapter 2.

A 6.　**A.** false　**B.** false　**C.** false　**D.** true　**E.** false

Local anaesthesia also affects motor and autonomic fibres.

The acid environment in situations such as cutaneous abscesses inhibits the action of local anaesthetics.

Topical anaesthetics, for example, cutaneous creams and throat sprays are used ubiquitously.

Fundamentals of Surgical Practice Chapter 2.

A 7.　**A.** true　**B.** false　**C.** false　**D.** false　**E.** false

Pulse oximetry is also used routinely when patients are sedated (e.g. for endoscopy).

Patients may breathe spontaneously under general anaesthesia. This is only necessary when muscle relaxation is necessary (e.g. for abdominal surgery).

Bradycardia is treated with atropine.

Fundamentals of Surgical Practice Chapter 2.

Postoperative Management

Answers

A 1. **A.** true **B.** false **C.** true **D.** true **E.** true

Allergic reactions to blood transfusion may be mild urticaria through to generalised anaphylaxis.

Hyperkalaemia may develop due to leakage of potassium from stored red blood cells.

Transmission of hepatitis C virus is a recognised cause of subsequent development of cirrhosis.

Microaggregates may be responsible for the development of ARDS.

Haemolytic jaundice may result from lysis of transfused red blood cells.

Fundamentals of Surgical Practice Chapter 3.

A 2. **A.** true **B.** true **C.** false **D.** true **E.** true

Atelectasis is collapse of a group of alveoli or lung segment. Therefore gas exchange may be impaired. Unless adequately treated, atelectasis may predispose to chest infection.

Treatment of atelectasis consists of lung expansion and clearing of stagnant secretions. Adequate pain relief is crucial. Coughing, chest physiotherapy and the occasional use of mucolytic agents and tracheal suction successfully reverses atelectasis.

Fever within the first 48 h after surgery is usually caused by atelectasis.

Fibreoptic bronchoscopy is occasionally required.

Fundamentals of Surgical Practice Chapter 3.

A 3. **A.** false **B.** true **C.** false **D.** false **E.** false

It is unnecessary and probably unwise to administer potassium during the first 24 h postoperatively.

Insensible fluid losses usually average 600–900 ml daily. This may, however, be increased to 1500 ml by hypermetabolism, hyperventilation or fever.

Blood should be administered if the haematocrit falls below 30%.

Daily fluid requirement for the first few postoperative days may supply limited calories, however supplemental nutrition should only be considerd if a more prolonged period of inadequate oral intake is anticipated.

A central venous pressure of between 2 and 10 cm H_2O is normal and fluid replacement need not be increased if the other vital signs, such as pulse rate, blood pressure and urinary output are adequate.

Fundamentals of Surgical Practice Chapter 3.

A 4. **A.** true **B.** true **C.** false **D.** true **E.** false

The most common site of intra-abdominal abscess formation is below the diaphragm.

Tachycardia is the earliest sign of hypovolaemia, followed by hypotension when compensatory mechanisms are overwhelmed.

Ischaemic injury confined to the renal medulla is reversible, however, cortical necrosis is often irreversible.

Fundamentals of Surgical Practice Chapter 3.

A 5. **A.** false **B.** false **C.** true **D.** false **E.** true

Epidural anaesthesia usually remains in situ for 3–4 days and may mask early reactionary haemorrhage presenting with hypotension and silent peritonism. Secondary haemorrhage usually presents at 7–10 days after operation and therefore should not be masked by an epidural.

Nasogastric suction does not prevent postoperative intestinal ileus but is often used to treat the complications of an ileus.

Open drainage increases the risk of septic complications.

Fundamentals of Surgical Practice Chapter 3.

A 6. **A.** true **B.** true **C.** true **D.** true **E.** true

Subphrenic abscess is a potentially serious complication with a mortality rate of up to 20%. Percutaneous or surgical drainage combined with intravenous antibiotic administration is mandatory.

Low grade pyrexia on the first or second postoperative day may be secondary to pulmonary atelectasis and the same condition 4–7 days postoperatively may be secondary to a deep venous thrombosis.

Pyrexia during or after blood transfusion may be due to release of white blood cell antigens or due to a haemolytic transfusion reaction.

Fundamentals of Surgical Practice Chapter 3.

A 7. **A.** true **B.** false **C.** true **D.** false **E.** false

Acute renal failure is reported to occur in approximately 8–10% of jaundiced patients undergoing surgical intervention, although the incidence of postoperative renal dysfunction appears to be reducing with more aggressive preoperative fluid resuscitation and volume loading.

Deep venous thrombosis after varicose vein surgery is very rare.

Hyperglycaemia, high lactate levels and a prolonged prothrombin time following liver resection for colorectal metastases may indicate impaired hepatic reserve and if the values do not settle may progress to hepatic failure.

Chvostek's sign and Trousseau's sign are features of hypocalcaemia.

Hypocalcaemia is rare following thyroid lobectomy, but may occur following subtotal or total thyroidectomy if there is associated damage to the parathyroid glands.

Urinary retention is more common following inguinal hernia repair.

Fundamentals of Surgical Practice Chapter 3.

Nutritional Support — Answers

A 1. **A.** true **B.** true **C.** false **D.** true **E.** false

Other biochemical markers include transferrin and retinol binding protein.

The triceps skin-fold thickness is an anthropometric measurement as is the mid arm muscle circumference.

Handgrip strength is a dynamometric method to assess patients' nutritional status and to assess for protein energy malnutrition.

Fundamentals of Surgical Practice Chapter 4.

A 2. **A.** true **B.** true **C.** true **D.** false **E.** false

Low serum albumin contributes to peripheral oedema and this is a feature of severe malnutrition.

Koilonychia is associated with iron deficiency but is not a feature of severe malnutrition.

Fundamentals of Surgical Practice Chapter 4.

A 3. **A.** false **B.** true **C.** true **D.** true **E.** false

Enteral nutrition modifies the antibacterial host defences, blunts the hypermetabolic response to trauma, maintains gut mucosal mass and reduces the incidence of bacterial translocation.

Enteral nutrition maintains gut mucosal gut barrier function as it supplies enterocytes with their main source of nutrition.

For many critically ill patients including those following abdominal surgery, the gastrointestinal tract is an appropriate and important route for nutritional support, as long as there is no evidence of bowel dysfunction, manifest by abdominal distension, vomiting and large volume naso-gastric aspirate. Small bowel digestive and absorptive function is maintained in the post-operative period after abdominal surgery and therefore enteral nutrition may be safely administered immediately even in the presence of a newly fashioned anastomosis.

Enteral nutrition should be considered the first choice of feeding for patients with severe head injuries and should be commenced early as aggressive nutritional support confers benefit on outcome.

There are fewer septic complications in enterally fed patients compared with TPN fed patients.

Fundamentals of Surgical Practice Chapter 4.

A 4. **A.** true **B.** false **C.** false **D.** true **E.** true

For most adult patients 14–16 gms of nitrogen/24 h is required.

Approximately 1.5 g protein/day are required.

Fundamentals of Surgical Practice Chapter 4.

A 5. **A.** true **B.** true **C.** false **D.** true **E.** true

In general, enteral feeding can be given to patients with paralytic ileus. However, if there is evidence of mechanical bowel obstruction, enteral feeding is contraindicated and TPN should be administered.

A specific complication of TPN, of multifactorial aetiology, is the development of hepatic dysfunction. This is characterised by elevated hepatic enzymes, intra-hepatic cholestasis and fatty infiltration of the liver. This is generally self-limiting and hepatic function returns to normal after cessation of TPN.

Fundamentals of Surgical Practice Chapter 4.

A 1. **A.** true **B.** true **C.** true **D.** true **E.** false

Temperature >38.4°C or <35.6°C is a characteristic of SIRS.

White cell count >1200 cells per ml or <4000 cells per ml is a characteristic of SIRS.

Respiratory rate >20/min is a characteristic of SIRS.

$PaCO_2$ <32 mmHg is a characteristic of SIRS.

Fundamentals of Surgical Practice Chapter 5.

A 2. **A.** false **B.** false **C.** true **D.** true **E.** false

Small intestinal stasis promotes the overgrowth of pathogenic bacteria in the gastrointestinal tract.

Secretion of IgA prevents intestinal bacterial overgrowth.

Blind loops of bowel promote overgrowth of pathogenic bacteria.

Fundamentals of Surgical Practice Chapter 5.

A 3. **A.** false **B.** true **C.** true **D.** true **E.** false

Oropharyngeal colonisation in critically ill patients is due to lack of mastication and salivation rather than increased mouth breathing.

H_2 antagonists neutralise gastric acid allowing bacteria to colonise in the stomach.

The presence of a nasogastric tube leads to a loss of lower oesophageal sphincter competence, allowing bacteria to ascend from the stomach to the upper airways.

The presence of an endotracheal tube allows environmental organisms to gain entry into the airways and lungs thus, predisposing to nosocomial pneumonia.

The cough reflex is impaired in patients with a decreased level of consciousness and this is a predisposing factor for nosocomial pneumonia rather than an impaired gag reflex.

Fundamentals of Surgical Practice Chapter 5.

A 4. **A.** true **B.** true **C.** true **D.** true **E.** true

The presence of organisms or their breakdown products i.e. endotoxin, peptidoglycans and teichoic acid may initiate the release of mediators responsible for the inflammatory response in sepsis. Pro-inflammatory cytokines such as tumour necrosis factor (TNF), interleukin-6 (IL-6), IL-8 and platelet activating factors (PAF) are released by macrophages and other immune cells. These polypeptides have multiple biological activities although many of their individual effects remain a mystery.

In addition to proinflammatory cytokines a number of anti-inflammatory cytokines are also released in the presence of systemic endotoxaemia.

The release of pro-inflammatory cytokines may also lead to the activation of the arachidonic and complement cascades.

Fundamentals of Surgical Practice Chapter 5.

A 5. **A.** true **B.** true **C.** true **D.** true **E.** true

Other complications associated with surgery in patients with obstructive jaundice include renal dysfunction, bleeding problems, impaired wound healing and other septic complications.

Fundamentals of Surgical Practice Chapter 5.

A 6. **A.** false **B.** false **C.** true **D.** false **E.** true

Lung compliance is reduced in this syndrome due to the accumulation of interstitial fluid and alveolar oedema secondary to increased tissue permeability.

ARDS should be suspected if hypoxaemia persists despite increasing inspired oxygen concentration.

A patient with ARDS is often confused because of the hypoxaemia but encephalopathy refers to patients with liver failure.

Patients with ARDS are usually tachypnoeic and dyspnoeic.

Fundamentals of Surgical Practice Chapter 5.

A 7. **A.** true **B.** false **C.** false **D.** true **E.** true

Penicillins are bactericidal and act by disrupting the peptidoglycan of the bacteria cell wall.

Ampicillin is commonly used for infections due to *E. coli*, proteus and *Haemophilus influenzae* but is ineffective against pseudomonas.

Though suggested to be effective as monotherapeutic agents, cephalosporans are normally used in conjunction with an aminoglycoside and metronidazole to provide adequate cover for enteric organisms and anerobes in intra-abdominal sepsis.

The most feared side effects of aminoglycosides are nephrotoxicity and ototoxicity.

Fundamentals of Surgical Practice Chapter 5.

A 8. **A.** true **B.** true **C.** false **D.** false **E.** true

Patients who are infected with HIV, HBV or HCV need not be isolated unless they are actively bleeding or likely to bleed, such as those with oesophageal varices.

Patients with diarrhoea and vomiting and any of the above infections should be isolated.

Unless patients with HIV, HBV or HCV have urinary or faecal incontinence, they need not be isolated for a simple urinary tract infection.

Patients with surgical drains or open wounds should be isolated.

Fundamentals of Surgical Practice Chapter 5.

Surgical Techniques & Technology

Answers

A 1. **A.** true **B.** false **C.** true **D.** true **E.** false

Local infiltration of anaesthetic agent is commonly used to manipulate wrist fractures.

Zadek's procedure involves excision of the nail of the great toe. Adrenaline should be avoided because of the risk of inducing digital artery spasm and toe ischaemia.

A nerve block combined with a field block around the ilioinguinal and iliohypogastric nerves as they lie between the internal and external oblique muscles about 2 cm medial to the anterior superior iliac spine provides good anaesthesia for repair of an inguinal hernia.

Local anaesthesia is useful for painless insertion of central venous catheters.

A Seton suture is used in the management of anal fistulas. This requires insertion of a probe through the fistulous tract under general anaesthesia and is not a suitable procedure for local anaesthesia.

Fundamentals of Surgical Practice Chapter 6.

A 2. **A.** true **B.** true **C.** false **D.** true **E.** false

Diathermy is a high-frequency alternating current which produces heat, not by the effect of electrical resistance but by oscillation of the ions in the tissues. In bipolar form, current passes between two closely adjacent electrodes so that the current does not pass through the body of the patient. There is a risk of thrombosis of the dorsal vein of the penis using monopolar diathermy during circumcision.

Grade IV liver injuries are major lacerations or significant haematomas of the liver which would not be adequately controlled by diathermy and require more extensive surgical intervention.

If the large plate of a monopolar diathermy does not make good contact, or its lead is broken, current can flow through alternative routes, including metal in contact with the patient, and cause burns.

Neodynium yttrium aluminium garnet (NdYAG) is a laser medium rather than diathermy modality. It can, however, be transmitted through optic fibres to destroy lesions in the gastrointestinal tract.

Fundamentals of Surgical Practice Chapter 6.

A 3. **A.** true **B.** true **C.** false **D.** true **E.** false

Serotonin and histamine release by mast cells result in dilatation of venules and increase vascular permeability.

Growth factors stimulate the proliferation of fibroblasts. Cytokines act as chemoattractants and activators of white blood cells.

Wound contracture is due to shortening of collagen fibres.

Vitamin A deficiency retards epithelialisation and collagen synthesis.

There is no evidence to support the concept that nutrients improve or speed healing.

Fundamentals of Surgical Practice Chapter 6.

A 4. **A.** false **B.** true **C.** true **D.** true **E.** true

Ultraviolet light has been shown in experimental and clinical studies to promote wound healing.

Wound healing is impaired in patients with obstructive jaundice. This may be due to the presence of endotoxaemia and/or concomitant factors such as poor nutritional status or malignancy.

Neoplasia is associated with poor wound healing.

Previous exposure to ionising radiation causes permanently reduced vascularity in exposed tissues which impairs wound healing.

Infection is a potent inhibitor of healing.

Fundamentals of Surgical Practice Chapter 6.

A 5. **A.** false **B.** false **C.** true **D.** true **E.** true

The accepted incidence of wound infections in clean wounds is approximately 2%.

Shaving the operative site 24h prior to surgery increases the wound infection rate and therefore should be performed immediately prior to surgery.

A prolonged preoperative stay increases the risk of nosocomial infections.

Many enzymes are zinc-dependent.

Fundamentals of Surgical Practice Chapter 6.

A 6. **A.** false **B.** true **C.** true **D.** true **E.** false

Adults with 15% and children with 10% of body surface burned need to be admitted to hospital.

Longitudinal incisions (escarotomy) should be performed following circumferential deep burns of the thorax to avoid restriction of chest movement and impaired respiratory function.

Superficial burns are painful, full thickness burns are painless and needle pricks cannot be felt, whereas partial thickness burns are often painless but needle pricks can usually be felt.

Burn injuries to the head and neck are more frequently associated with concomitant smoke inhalation and respiratory complications and therefore are associated with higher morbidity and mortality rates.

Fundamentals of Surgical Practice Chapter 6.

A 7.   **A.** true   **B.** true   **C.** false   **D.** true   **E.** true

Nutritional requirements in severely burned patients may double.

Both cellular and humoral immune function are depressed.

Hyponatraemia may occur as there is loss of sodium from the burn oedema, failure of the sodium pump and marked ADH secretion.

Hypoalbuminaemia may occur due to loss from the burn and impaired liver synthesis.

Impaired gut barrier function associated with burn injuries may be associated with an increased incidence of subsequent septic complications.

Fundamentals of Surgical Practice Chapter 6.

A 8.   **A.** true   **B.** false   **C.** true   **D.** false   **E.** false

Early enteral nutrition may improve gut barrier function and reduce bacterial and endotoxin translocation and thereby potentially reduce subsequent septic complications.

Administration of broad-spectrum antibiotics will increase antibiotic-resistant bacterial strains and therefore antibiotics should only be administered for significant sepsis.

Dressings should absorb wound exudate and should be changed only when the exudate threatens to soak through the dressings.

Premature surgical intervention before contracture maturation increases the number of procedures required and results in a worse aesthetic result.

Fundamentals of Surgical Practice Chapter 6.

Trauma: General Principles of Management

Answers

A 1. **A.** false **B.** false **C.** true **D.** true **E.** false

The presence of hypovolaemic shock suggests there may be other injuries as facial injuries rarely result in significant blood loss.

At all times, a patent airway must be maintained. The casualty should be positioned semi-upright and have an oropharyngeal airway in place.

Significant swelling and oedema can develop and lead to obstruction of the airway: this may prevent insertion of an endotracheal tube and may necessitate performing a surgical cricothyroidotomy.

Airway patency should be achieved with cervical spine control at all times. It should therefore be considered in association with airway control and excluded after securing a definitive airway.

Fundamentals of Surgical Practice Chapter 7.

A 2. **A.** false **B.** false **C.** false **D.** false **E.** false

Tourniquets should not be used because they crush tissues and cause distal ischaemia. External blood loss should be minimised by direct manual pressure.

Airway patency is important, however, adequate ventilation and gas exchange also requires adequate function of the lungs, chest wall and diaphragm.

Urinary catheterisation is contraindicated in patients with suspected urethral transection.

A normal lateral cervical spine X-ray is reassuring but does not exclude a cervical spine injury.

Contraindications for nasotracheal intubation are apnoea, severe midfacial fractures or where there is suspicion of a basilar skull fracture.

Fundamentals of Surgical Practice Chapter 7.

A **3.** **A.** true **B.** false **C.** false **D.** true **E.** true

Blood pressure is maintained until decompensation occurs, usually when >1500 ml of blood has been lost.

Tissue perfusion of the vital organs is maintained until decompensation occurs.

Heart rate is a poor indicator of haemorrhage, however, tachycardia may develop as the patient decompensates.

A patient can usually tolerate up to 1500 ml blood loss before decompensation occurs.

Fundamentals of Surgical Practice Chapter 7.

A **4.** **A.** true **B.** true **C.** true **D.** true **E.** false

Increased intracranial pressure may cause a reflex increase in systemic arterial blood pressure in order to maintain cerebral perfusion. This phenomenon is known as Cushing's reflex.

Diffuse axonal injury occurs when deceleration forces cause a shearing injury to brain tissue and may not be apparent on CT scan.

Retention of carbon dioxide may be due to a depressed level of consciousness. It results in cerebral vasodilation and will tend to increase cerebral blood volume.

Severe head injury is defined as a Glasgow Coma Score of 8 or less.

Fundamentals of Surgical Practice Chapter 7.

A **5.** **A.** true **B.** false **C.** true **D.** false **E.** false

Patients with exsanguinating, penetrating precordial injuries who arrive pulseless but with myocardial electrical activity may be candidates for emergency department thoracotomy. Emergency department thoracotomy for patients with blunt thoracic injuries, in whom there is no electrical cardiac activity, is rarely effective.

If 1500 ml blood is immediately evacuated on insertion of a chest drain, it is highly likely that the patient will require a thoracotomy.

Aortic transection may be suspected from widening of the mediastinum on chest X-ray, however, a definitive diagnosis is made by arch aortography.

Appropriate management of a patient with a flail chest segment includes adequate ventilatory support and analgesia. Some patients require a short period of endotracheal intubation and ventilation.

Fundamentals of Surgical Practice Chapter 7.

A 6. **A.** false **B.** true **C.** true **D.** false **E.** true

Stab wounds to the back should be managed conservatively if possible. Kidneys avulsed from their vascular pedicle following blunt trauma may need to be removed. Abdominal gunshot wounds should be treated by routine laparotomy because of the high (>90%) incidence of visceral damage.

Many stab wounds can be managed conservatively, however indications for laparotomy are if there are signs of shock, peritonitis or visceral protrusion.

A liver laceration and evidence of free intra-abdominal blood on CT scan is not a definitive indication for laparotomy. Previously, many patients underwent an unnecessary laparotomy as the bleeding had stopped by the time of surgical intervention. Therefore, many of these patients can be treated conservatively if they remain haemodynamically stable.

Fundamentals of Surgical Practice Chapter 7.

A 7. **A.** false **B.** false **C.** true **D.** false **E.** true

Diagnostic peritoneal lavage (DPL) is more sensitive, but less specific, than CT scan for intraperitoneal bleeding.

DPL is positive if the red cell count is >100,000 RBCs/mm³ and if the white cell count is >500 WBCs/mm³.

An unstable patient with peritonism should undergo laparotomy without the delay in performing a DPL.

Fundamentals of Surgical Practice Chapter 7.

A 8.   **A.** true   **B.** true   **C.** true   **D.** false   **E.** false

Liver injuries in the UK are predominantly due to blunt trauma, which contrasts with studies in the United States, where penetrating trauma is more prevalent.

Hyperpyrexia is common following liver trauma and may be due to resorption of devitalised parenchyma and hepatocellular regeneration.

Anatomical resection is rarely indicated. Hepatotomy with direct suture ligation of bleeding vessels or resectional debridement utilising lines of injury rather than anatomical planes are more commonly applied techniques.

Perihepatic packing should be used rather than intrahepatic packing as the latter method tends to open up and may even extend liver lacerations. Perihepatic packing to achieve haemodynamic stability is important in the management of significant liver injuries prior to transfer of the patient to a specialist liver unit.

A 9.   **A.** false   **B.** true   **C.** false   **D.** false   **E.** false

100% oxygen should be administered if an inhalation injury is suspected.

One half of the estimated fluid requirement for the first 24 h should be administered over the first 8 h and the remainder over the next 16 h.

Prophylactic antibiotics are not indicated in the early postburn period. Antibiotics should be reserved for the treatment of infection.

Alkali burns are generally more serious than acid burns, because the alkali penetrates more deeply.

Fundamentals of Surgical Practice Chapter 7.

A **10.** **A.** true **B.** true **C.** false **D.** false **E.** false

Increased secretion of ADH results in increased water reabsorption in the renal tubules.

ACTH secretion from the pituitary gland is increased due to stimulation by corticotropin releasing factor (CRF) released from the hypothalamus.

Hyperglycaemia may result from increased glycogenolysis due to increased adrenaline secretion. In addition, glucose utilisation may be reduced because of inhibited insulin secretion.

Renin secretion is increased, which serves to conserve sodium (via angiotensin) at the expense of increased potassium loss.

Fundamentals of Surgical Practice Chapter 7.

A 1. **A.** false **B.** true **C.** true **D.** true **E.** true

Cardiac output is a function of stroke volume and heart rate.

Input from baroreceptors and chemoreceptors may alter cardiac output by altering the sympathetic and parasympathetic discharges to the heart.

Thermodilution is the most commonly used technique for measuring cardiac output in ICU.

Fundamentals of Surgical Practice Chapter 8.

A 2. **A.** false **B.** true **C.** false **D.** true **E.** false

Cardiac tamponade is due to accumulation of fluid or clot in the pericardial space and is not exacerbated by pulmonary disease. It results in a raised CVP and may be treated by pericardiocentesis.

Pulsus paradoxus is said to occur when there is a greater than normal fall in arterial pressure during inspiration and occurs with cardiac tamponade.

Fundamentals of Surgical Practice Chapter 8.

A 3. **A.** true **B.** false **C.** true **D.** false **E.** true

ARDS may occur after severe tissue trauma, Gram-negative septicaemia, massive blood transfusion or acute pancreatitis. It is associated with reduced lung compliance (stiff lungs).

Early clinical signs include tachypnoea, dyspnoea and hypoxaemia before the development of radiological signs.

Fundamentals of Surgical Practice Chapter 8.

A 4. **A.** true **B.** false **C.** true **D.** false **E.** true

Type III respiratory failure is caused by combined failure of oxygenation and ventilation and may be due to ARDS, asthma and COAD. If PO_2 >55 mmHg in room air, PCO_2 >50 mmHg or respiratory rate >40/min then artificial ventilation is indicated.

Artificial ventilation is best achieved with relatively high tidal volumes (12–15 ml/kg) at a relatively slow rate (8–12 breaths/min).

Prolonged mechanical ventilation will result in respiratory muscle wasting and dysfunction which may prolong weaning.

With total ventilator support, the patient is paralysed and unable to contribute to the work of breathing so as to avoid ventilator-induced lung injury. Partial ventilator support allows the patient to contribute to the work of breathing.

Fundamentals of Surgical Practice Chapter 8.

A 5. **A.** false **B.** false **C.** true **D.** true **E.** true

Often, no septic focus is present in SIRS. Organ dysfunction may result from the systemic inflammatory response syndrome.

Impairment of gut barrier function may lead to spread of bacteria and endotoxin from the gut (a process known as bacterial translocation) which may initiate, exacerbate or perpetuate the systemic inflammatory response syndrome.

In addition to pro-inflammatory mediators (such as TNF and IL-6) anti-inflammatory mediators (such as IL-4 and IL-10) are released. A balance is required between these mediators to maintain homeostasis and facilitate recovery of the patient.

Fundamentals of Surgical Practice Chapter 8.

A 6. **A.** true **B.** false **C.** false **D.** false **E.** false

Renal impairment is defined as a urinary output of <800 ml/24 h. Acute renal failure is defined as a urinary output of <400 ml/24 h in the presence of a rising urea and creatinine. It may result in hyperkalaemia.

Acute renal failure can be minimized by treatment with dopamine administered at a rate of 0.5–3 mg/kg/min.

Haemodialysis can rapidly clear urea and creatinine but is associated with large shifts between the various fluid compartments. Thus it may be risky in critically ill patients who may be haemodynamically unstable. It is thus mainly used for patients with chronic renal failure. Continuous veno-venous haemofiltration is now the procedure of choice for renal support of critically ill patients.

Fundamentals of Surgical Practice Chapter 8.

A 7. **A.** false **B.** false **C.** false **D.** true **E.** true

Hypertension due to raised intracranial pressure may be associated with acute liver failure.

Hypoglycaemia may result from impairment of gluconeogenesis and depletion of glycogen stores.

Hyponatraemia may result from water retention and haemodilution.

Fundamentals of Surgical Practice Chapter 8.

Intensive Care

Answers

Principles of Cancer Management

Answers

A 1.   **A.** false   **B.** false   **C.** true   **D.** true   **E.** false

Aflatoxin is a possible cofactor to hepatitis B virus for liver cancer, but not pancreatic cancer.

Beta-carotene, found in green-yellow vegetables such as pumpkin, carrot, spinach, green lettuce and green asparagus, may protect against the development of stomach, lung and breast cancer.

Epstein-Barr virus is associated with nasopharyngeal cancer and Burkitt's lymphoma.

Liver cancer is associated with cirrhosis due to hepatitis B and hepatitis C.

Human papilloma virus is associated with genital and cervical cancer.

Fundamentals of Surgical Practice   Chapter 9.

A 2.   **A.** true   **B.** false   **C.** true   **D.** true   **E.** true

Specificity is the reciprocal of the false positive rate.

Fundamentals of Surgical Practice   Chapter 9.

A 3.   **A.** false   **B.** true   **C.** true   **D.** false   **E.** true

Calcitonin is associated with medullary carcinoma of the thyroid.

Alpha-feto protein is associated with hepatocellular carcinoma but not liver metastases.

Carcinoembryonic antigen is useful in monitoring treatment of carcinoma of the colon and rectum, either to determine the completeness of surgical removal or to predict impending clinical relapse during follow-up. It is insufficiently sensitive to use as a screening test.

A 4.   **A.** false   **B.** true   **C.** true   **D.** false   **E.** true

Brachytherapy is the application of radiotherapy within or near a tumour.

Anoxic cells require greater doses of radiation to destroy compared to well-oxygenated cells. Therefore hyperbaric oxygen has been administered as a radiosensitiser.

Photodynamic therapy utilises a combination of light and photosensitising drugs to treat accessible deposits of cancer. It has been used as palliation for advanced or metastatic cancers and as an adjuvant to surgery for mesothelioma and brain tumours. Recently it has been used as primary treatment for lung cancers, to eradicate multiple skin cancers in the basal cell naevus syndrome, and to treat premalignant lesions such as Barrett's oesophagus.

Neoadjuvant therapy is the administration of systemic therapy before local treatment, reducing the bulk of the primary tumour before surgery or radiotherapy.

There are pharmacological sanctuaries where drugs can fail to penetrate (e.g. within the CSF compartments due to the blood-brain barrier).

Fundamentals of Surgical Practice Chapter 9.

A 5.   **A.** true   **B.** true   **C.** false   **D.** false   **E.** false

Pleomorphism is the occurrence of cells of different size and shape and is characteristic of malignancy.

Anaplasia is a term used to describe the lack of resemblence of malignant tumour to the normal tissue of origin.

Metaplasia describes change in mature cells in a tissue to a form abnormal to that tissue, but does not imply the cells are malignant or invasive.

Reactive hyperplasia is not characteristic of malignancy.

Ulceration is not pathognomonic for malignancy and can be seen in benign conditions, such as peptic ulceration.

Fundamentals of Surgical Practice Chapter 9.

A 6. **A.** true **B.** true **C.** true **D.** false **E.** false

Hormones such as ACTH or ADH may be secreted by small cell anaplastic tumours of the lung.

This is well recognised and the ovarian lesions are known as Krukenberg tumours.

Right-sided colon cancers rarely present with obstruction, but usually present with altered bowel habit, anaemia or weight loss. Left-sided colonic cancers more commonly present with intestinal obstruction as the lumen is narrower and the bowel contents are more solid in nature.

Carcinoma of the tail of the pancreas usually presents at an advanced stage and can rarely be resected. Carcinoma of the head of the pancreas may present earlier with obstructive jaundice, however, only 10–20% of these patients will be suitable for potentially curative resection.

Fundamentals of Surgical Practice Chapter 9.

A 7. **A.** true **B.** true **C.** false **D.** false **E.** true

CEA is not specific for colorectal carcinoma, but may be used to monitor the effect of surgical resection of liver metastases and to detect occult tumour recurrence.

Hepatocellular carcinoma expresses AFP but cholangiocarcinoma does not.

Seminomas do not secrete HCG, however, testicular teratomas may express this tumour marker.

Fundamentals of Surgical Practice Chapter 9.

A. true   **B.** true   **C.** false   **D.** false   **E.** true

Patients with familial adenomatous polyposis invariably develop colorectal carcinoma in early adulthood unless colectomy is performed.

It is reported that the risk of developing an oesophageal adenocarcinoma in patients with Barretts oesophagus is increased 30–40 times that of the general population.

Although keratoacanthoma contains cells which resemble those of a squamous carcinoma, the lesion is not a premalignant condition.

Gastric fundic gland polyps are considered as hamartomatous lesions and there is no evidence of an increased risk of gastric cancer. Neoplastic gastric polyps are referred to as adenomas and histologically have a tubular configuration. The risk of malignant transformation is reported to occur in up to 40% of those adenomas greater than 2 cm in size.

Postcricoid dysphagia due to oesophageal mucosal webs associated with iron deficiency anaemia is known as Plummer-Vinson or Patterson-Kelly-Brown syndrome and is associated with a high incidence of oesophageal tumours.

Fundamentals of Surgical Practice Chapter 9.

Ethics, Legal Aspects & Assessment of Effectiveness

Answers

A 1. **A.** false   **B.** false   **C.** false   **D.** true   **E.** false

The age for the ability to give consent in British law is 18 years.

In Law, no person is capable of giving or withholding consent for another adult. In cases where patients are mentally or physically incapable of giving consent, the consent is given by the senior doctor caring for the patient and is undertaken on a specific type of consent form.

Consent generally does apply to all aspects of operative treatment but the patient can specifically state whether or not there is a particular aspect of treatment they do not wish to give consent to, e.g. a Jehovah's Witness can consent to an operation but refuse specifically to receive a blood transfusion.

If a parent refuses essential treatment for a child and the doctor feels that this is not in the child's best interest, the legal situation is that the child is not in the position to make an informed choice and if the doctor feels that the person acting on its behalf is not making a correct decision, the doctor can apply for the child to be made a ward of court.

Fundamentals of Surgical Practice Chapter 10.

A 1. **A.** true **B.** true **C.** true **D.** false **E.** true

PDGF is an example of several growth factors which promote cellular proliferation and the inflammatory response.

Tumour necrosis factors Alpha and Beta are potent pro-inflammatory cytokines and are released early during an inflammatory response.

There are many interleukins – some have pro and some have anti-inflammatory effects. The best known pro-inflammatory interleukin mediators is IL-6.

Erythropoietin is a glycoprotein hormone which regulates red blood cell formation.

Leucotrienes are products of arachidonic acid metabolism.

Fundamentals of Surgical Practice Chapter 11.

A 2. **A.** true **B.** false **C.** false **D.** false **E.** false

Excess iron is stored in the liver.

Red blood cells for transfusion can be stored for up to 35 days at 4°C.

DIC results in a decreased platelet count and increased fibrin degradation products.

DIC results in an increased bleeding time.

Fundamentals of Surgical Practice Chapter 11.

A 3.   **A.** false   **B.** true   **C.** false   **D.** false   **E.** false

Splenectomy results in thrombocytosis and an increased tendency to venous thrombosis.

Splenectomy results in an increase in infection and vaccinations against *Haemophylus influenzae*, pnuemococcus and meningococcus are recommended. In addition, long-term antibiotic therapy is recommended to reduce the risk of overwhelming post-splenectomy infection (OPSI).

Idiopathic thrombocytopaenic purpura is a rare indication for splenectomy. Common indications include trauma and lymphoma.

Trauma is not an absolute indication for splenectomy in haemodynamically stable patients, particularly children and splenic trauma can be managed conservatively with careful haemodynamic follow up. If laparotomy is necessary a repair procedure (splenorrhaphy) may be feasible rather than a splenectomy.

Implantation of diced splenic tissue in the omentum after splenectomy can result in viable splenic tissue which maintains a blood supply and is apparent on post-operative splenic scanning. However, such tissue has never been shown to be functional from an immunological point of view and the procedure of implantation of diced splenic tissue has largely been abandoned.

Fundamentals of Surgical Practice   Chapter 11.

A 1. **A.** false **B.** true **C.** true **D.** false **E.** false

The transpyloric plane is an imaginary line running between the tips of the ninth costal cartilages and corresponds to the level of L1 posteriorly. The superior mesenteric vein joins the splenic vein behind the pancreas to form the portal vein.

Fundamentals of Surgical Practice Chapter 12.

A 2. **A.** false **B.** true **C.** true **D.** true **E.** false

Oesophageal pH monitoring should be performed 5 cm above the level of the gastro-oesophageal junction.

Pre- and post-operative measurements of oesophageal pH confirms the effectiveness of anti-reflux surgery in patients with GORD.

Zollinger-Ellison Syndrome is diagnosed by a raised fasting gastrin level.

Fundamentals of Surgical Practice Chapter 12.

A 3. **A.** false **B.** true **C.** true **D.** false **E.** true

An ileostomy typically produces approximately 500 ml small intestinal content per day which has a high sodium content.

If a significant length of terminal ileum has been removed, vitamin B12 deficiency may be a feature in the longer term.

The desired design is a spout ileostomy to avoid retraction and facilitate skin care.

An ileostomy is associated with an increased incidence of gallstones and renal calculi which may be due to excess loss of fluid via the ileostomy which is normally reabsorbed in the large bowel.

Fundamentals of Surgical Practice Chapter 12.

A 4. **A.** true **B.** false **C.** false **D.** false **E.** true

If nasogastric drainage is anticipated for a prolonged period, a gastrostomy may be fashioned in the stomach as prolonged drainage via an NG tube may be uncomfortable for the patient and may be associated with oesophageal reflux and benign stricture formation.

A PEG tube is poor palliation for malignant oesophageal obstruction and is rarely indicated in this condition. Palliation using plastic tubes or metal self-expanding stents are more commonly used.

A liquid stool from a proximal colostomy makes its management more difficult than a colostomy formed in the left colon.

There is no evidence that creating a defunctioning loop ileostomy reduces the anastomotic leak rate following a low anterior resection. The advantage is that should a leak occur, the bowel is defunctioned preventing faecal spillage and peritoneal contamination.

Enteral feeding has been shown to help maintain gut barrier function by preventing intestinal villous atrophy and thereby reduce the incidence of postoperative nosocomial infections following major abdominal surgery.

Fundamentals of Surgical Practice Chapter 12.

A 5. **A.** false **B.** false **C.** false **D.** false **E.** false

Assessment of gastrointestinal and urological injuries is part of the secondary survey.

Localised peritonism in the left upper quadrant may indicate an underlying splenic injury, however, many of these injuries can be safely managed conservatively if the patient is haemodynamically stable and can be closely monitored in an appropriate setting.

Plain abdominal X-rays are generally unhelpful following blunt abdominal trauma. Free gas under the diaphragm in an erect chest X-ray indicates a ruptured hollow viscus.

Patients with generalised peritonitis and persistent hypotension require immediate laparotomy for control of haemorrhage. CT scanning wastes valuable time and may put the patient's life at risk – it should not be undertaken in this situation.

Many abdominal stab wounds can be managed conservatively and omentum protruding through an abdominal wound is not a definite indication for surgical exploration. If the patient is haemodynamically stable and has no signs of peritonism, further radiological evaluation should be perfomed and the patient monitored closely.

Fundamentals of Surgical Practice Chapter 12.

A 6. A. false **B.** false **C.** false **D.** true **E.** true

The spleen is the most frequently injured solid intra-abdominal organ following blunt trauma.

Gun shot wounds require exploratory laparotomy, however, stab wounds can often be managed conservatively if the patient remains haemodynamically stable.

Perihepatic packing is extremely useful in the treatment of liver injuries when the patient is haemodynamically unstable and can be left for 24–48 h until the overall condition of the patient improves before being removed. However, packs should not be inserted into liver lacerations as this may extend the laceration and exacerbate bleeding.

Fundamentals of Surgical Practice Chapter 12.

A 7. A. true **B.** false **C.** true **D.** true **E.** false

Meckel's diverticulum is a rare cause of acute abdominal pain. Although approximately 2% of the population have a Meckel's diverticulum, few patients develop acute symptoms.

Appendicitis accounts for approximately 25% of acute admissions for acute abdominal pain.

Mesenteric ischaemia is a rare cause of acute abdominal pain.

Fundamentals of Surgical Practice Chapter 12.

A 8. **A.** false **B.** true **C.** true **D.** true **E.** false

Pus should be drained percutaneously by insertion of a drain under radiological guidance.

Appendicitis may be secondary to an underlying caecal carcinoma and therefore careful evaluation of the caecum should be undertaken in elderly patients.

Delayed appendicectomy is not mandatory as the pathological process will result in fibrosis of the appendix. Therefore in young people in whom a caecal tumour is unlikely, no further surgical intervention may be required.

Fundamentals of Surgical Practice Chapter 12.

A 9. **A.** true **B.** false **C.** true **D.** false **E.** true

Laparoscopy is used increasingly to diagnose and treat acute conditions, such as appendicitis, especially in young females.

Diagnostic peritoneal lavage is useful to assess the need for surgical intervention in patients following blunt abdominal trauma but is rarely used to investigate patients with an acute abdomen. Only 10% of gallstones are radio-opaque and therefore approximately 90% will not be visualised on an abdominal X-ray. Ultrasonography is useful to differentiate many causes of an acute abdomen.

Serum amylase is useful to exclude acute pancreatitis as a cause of acute abdominal pain.

Fundamentals of Surgical Practice Chapter 12.

A 10. **A.** false **B.** true **C.** false **D.** true **E.** true

Clinical examination in acute cholecystitis may reveal a tachycardia. Deep palpation in the right hypochondrium when the patient inspires deeply may be painful (Murphy's sign).

Pain often starts in the epigastrium as the gallbladder is a foregut structure and then localises in the right hypochondrium. Midgut structures classically present with initial periumbilical pain.

Formation of a cholecystostomy by insertion of a percutaneous drain may allow dramatic resolution of symptoms and may be lifesaving in elderly unfit patients.

Fundamentals of Surgical Practice Chapter 12.

A **11.** **A.** true **B.** true **C.** true **D.** false **E.** false

Idiopathic pancreatitis accounts for up to 20% of cases of acute pancreatitis.

Serum amylase will be diagnostic in 85–90% of cases, however, in patients presenting early or late in the course of the disease, the amylase peak, which is only sustained for 12–24 h, may be missed.

Pancreatic carcinoma is a rare cause of pancreatitis. Pancreatic necrosis demonstrated on CT scan is not a definite indication for surgical intervention. Necrosectomy is indicated if there is evidence of infected necrosis or the patient's clinical condition deteriorates with evidence of impending organ failure.

Cholecystectomy should be performed during the same hospital admission in patients presenting with gallstone induced pancreatitis.

Fundamentals of Surgical Practice Chapter 12.

A **12.** **A.** false **B.** true **C.** false **D.** true **E.** true

The commonest cause of small bowel obstruction is intra-abdominal adhesions.

Metabolic alkalosis may be associated with vomiting, and metabolic acidosis may be associated with intestinal infarction. Excessive vomiting may cause hypokalaemia.

Alimentary System

Answers

Gallstone ileus implies the passage of a large gallstone into the intestine via a biliary-enteric fistula which allows gas to pass into the biliary system.

Fundamentals of Surgical Practice Chapter 12.

A **13.** **A.** true **B.** true **C.** true **D.** false **E.** true

Endotoxaemia due to impaired gut barrier function and impaired host immune function are implicated in the development of these complications in jaundiced patients.

Silvery stools may be due to absence of bile salts in the gastrointestinal tract and some bleeding from the periampullary lesion.

Only 10–20% of Klatskin tumours (hilar cholangiocarcinoma) are suitable for major surgical resection. The majority of patients are palliated by insertion of an endoprosthesis.

Causes of obstructive jaundice following laparoscopic cholecystectomy include retained gallstones or bile duct injury.

Fundamentals of Surgical Practice Chapter 12.

A **14.** **A.** false **B.** false **C.** false **D.** false **E.** false

Recurrent obstruction and infection in the biliary tree due to gallstones may result in secondary biliary cirrhosis. Primary biliary cirrhosis is an autoimmune condition.

A mucocele of the gallbladder will not develop if the level of obstruction of the biliary tree is above the level of the cystic duct.

Gallstones of the diameter required to cause a gallstone ileus do not pass through the Sphincter of Oddi, but rather pass through a fistula between the gallbladder and the duodenum or small intestine.

A gallstone impacted at Hartman's pouch rarely causes obstructive jaundice.

Contrast in the venous system must be conjugated to bilirubin and excreted in the bile to outline the biliary system.

Fundamentals of Surgical Practice Chapter 12.

A **15.** **A.** true **B.** true **C.** true **D.** true **E.** false

Head injury may result in stress ulceration or erosions known as Cushings ulcers.

Excess production of gastrin from a gastrinoma in the Zollinger-Ellsion syndrome may produce multiple refractory peptic ulcers.

Bile reflux may cause damage to the gastric mucosa.

Peptic ulceration is associated with high intragastric acidity and low pH.

Fundamentals of Surgical Practice Chapter 12.

A **16.** **A.** true **B.** true **C.** false **D.** true **E.** true

Antibiotics commonly used to erradicate *Helicobacter pylori* include metronidazole, amoxycillin and clarithromycin.

Prostaglandin antagonists are associated with peptic ulceration.

Several surgical techniques are available with vagotomy and gastrojejunostomy often undertaken in patients with pyloric stenosis.

Fundamentals of Surgical Practice Chapter 12.

A **17.** **A.** true **B.** true **C.** true **D.** true **E.** true

An increased risk of oesophageal malignancy is thought to be due to stasis of food in the distended oesophagus.

Temporary relief of symptoms has been demonstrated following injection of Botulinum toxin at the level of the lower oesophageal sphincter. Other management options include hydrostatic dilation and Heller's cardiomyotomy.

Fundamentals of Surgical Practice Chapter 12.

A **18.** **A.** true   **B.** true   **C.** true   **D.** false   **E.** true

The inguinal ligament, inferior epigastric vessels and the lateral border of the rectus abdominus form the boundaries of Hasselbach's triangle.

Indirect inguinal hernias enter the deep inguinal ring lateral to the inferior epigastric vessels and are more likely to develop complications because of their narrower neck.

Fundamentals of Surgical Practice Chapter 12.

A **19.** **A.** false   **B.** false   **C.** true   **D.** true   **E.** false

Inguinal hernias are commoner than femoral hernias in females.

Due to the tight ligamentous ring around the neck of the sac, femoral herniae frequently become strangulated.

Fundamentals of Surgical Practice Chapter 12.

A **20.** **A.** false   **B.** false   **C.** true   **D.** true   **E.** true

Patients with oesophageal carcinoma rarely present with bleeding; the principle symptom is dysphagia.

Although the incidence of adenocarcinomas is rising, squamous cell carcinoma is still the commonest type of oesophageal malignancy.

Barrett's metaplasia is a premalignant condition and predisposes to the development of oesophageal adenocarcinoma. Barrett's oesophagus is usually regarded as a consequence of chronic gastro-oesophageal reflux and is thought to increase the risk of developing an adenocarcinoma by 30–40 times that of the general population.

The lymphatic drainage of the lower third of the oesophagus includes the coeliac trunk lymph nodes.

Approximately two thirds of patients are unresectable at presentation and can be palliated by endoscopic intubation with a variety of plastic stents or expandable metal stents.

Fundamentals of Surgical Practice Chapter 12.

A 21. A. false **B.** true **C.** true **D.** false **E.** true

Low socio-economic class is a risk factor for gastric cancer.

The risk of developing cancer after previous partial gastrectomy is thought to be approximately twice that of the control population. Those who are most at risk have undergone surgery before the age of 40 and the cancer commonly develops 15–20 years after partial gastrectomy.

Blood group A is associated with gastric cancer.

Fundamentals of Surgical Practice Chapter 12.

A 22. A. true **B.** true **C.** false **D.** true **E.** true

Linitis plastica describes a diffuse involvement of the stomach by tumour.

Troisier's sign is a palpable malignant left supraclavicular lymph node (Virchow's node).

Transcoelemic spread to the ovaries is known as Krukenberg's tumours.

Migratory thrombophlebitis is associated with gastric carcinoma.

Fundamentals of Surgical Practice Chapter 12.

A 23. A. false **B.** true **C.** false **D.** true **E.** false

The commonest presentation of pancreatic carcinoma is painless obstructive jaundice with dark urine, pale stools and pruritus, preceded by some weight loss. *Acanthosis nigricans* is an uncommon presentation.

Less than 20% of cases are resectable.

ERCP may demonstrate a complete occlusion of the distal common bile duct and the pancreatic duct giving a characteristic double duct sign.

Five year survival following Whipple pancreaticoduodenectomy is usually 5–10%, although there are some Japanese series with 5-year survival figures of 30–40%.

Fundamentals of Surgical Practice Chapter 12.

A 23. A. false   **B.** true   **C.** false   **D.** true   **E.** true

Colorectal cancer is the second most common malignancy in the Western world after lung cancer.

5–10% of patients with liver metastases are suitable for curative resection. Five year survival figures of 30–35% are reported in this group of patients.

Fundamentals of Surgical Practice Chapter 12.

A 1.   **A.** true   **B.** false   **C.** true   **D.** false   **E.** true

A 2.   **A.** false   **B.** true   **C.** true   **D.** false   **E.** true

Diabetes results in microangiopathy and chronic vascular disease.

Atheroma leads to chronic vascular disease but may predispose to acute embolism.

Arteritis may cause acute peripheral ischaemia with digital gangrene and also chronic vascular disease (e.g. Buerger's and Takayasu's disease).

Fundamentals of Surgical Practice Chapter 13.

A 3.   **A.** true   **B.** false   **C.** true   **D.** true   **E.** true

A 4.   **A.** true   **B.** true   **C.** false   **D.** false   **E.** false

A Doppler ultrasound detector may also be used instead of a stethoscope.

An index of 0.7 indicates moderate ischaemia. An index below 0.5 indicates severe ischaemia and is usually associated with rest pain.

Fundamentals of Surgical Practice Chapter 13.

A 5.   **A.** true   **B.** false   **C.** true   **D.** false   **E.** false

An aortic aneurysm >6 cm should be treated either using a prosthetic graft or by an endoluminal stent.

Destruction of the vessel media results in dissection by blood in this plane.

A false aneurysm develops when an artery is pierced and is surrounded by a haematoma which remains in continuity with the vessel lumen.

95% of aortic aneurysms occur below the level of the renal arteries.

Fundamentals of Surgical Practice Chapter 13.

A 6. **A.** false **B.** false **C.** true **D.** true **E.** true

Transluminal angioplasty is most successful in the iliac arteries and least successful below the popliteal arteries.

In the case of asymmetrical stenoses, the normal part of the arterial wall dilates without compression of the plaque.

Palmar and pedal hyperhidrosis and ischaemic cutaneous ulceration are all indications for sympathectomy: other indications include control of rest pain and vasospastic disorders.

Endarterectomy is used principally in the carotid, iliac and common femoral arteries. Its use in the aortoiliac region has largely been superceded by bypass grafting.

Fundamentals of Surgical Practice Chapter 13.

A 7. **A.** false **B.** false **C.** false **D.** false **E.** false

Primary or familial varicose veins occur in 10–25% of patients.

The majority of leg ulcers (70%) are associated with venous disease. Other commonly associated conditions include arterial disease (20%), hypertension (15–20%) and diabetes (5%).

Graduated compression is used in the vast majority of cases. Antibiotics may be indicated if there is surrounding cellulitis and dressing with desloughing agents may be indicated if slough is present.

Fundamentals of Surgical Practice Chapter 13.

Vascular Surgery

Answers

Endocrine Surgery — Answers

A 1. **A.** false **B.** true **C.** true **D.** true **E.** false

Reidel's lobe is associated with the liver and not the thyroid.

The thyroid gland is formed from an ectodermal downgrowth from the 1st and 2nd pharyngeal pouches and descends to a level just below the cricoid cartilage. This line of descent is known as the thyroglossal tract but embryological abnormalities include cell nests remaining in the line of the thyroglossal tract, which may result in the formation of a thyroglossal cyst.

Over descent may result in a retrosternal goitre.

On reaching its final position the thyroid divides into two lobes with a central isthmus. There may be agenesis of one lobe.

The foramen caecum of the tongue represents the embryological origin of the thyroid gland and is not a developmental abnormality.

Fundamentals of Surgical Practice Chapter 14.

A 2. **A.** true **B.** false **C.** false **D.** false **E.** false

Approximately 80 µg of free thyroxine is formed per day.

The majority of T3 in the tissues is formed by conversion of T4 to T3 at tissue level.

Thyroid secretion is controlled by TSH, which is released from the anterior pituitary gland.

The biological half-life of thyroxine is 6 days.

Fundamentals of Surgical Practice Chapter 14.

A 3. **A.** true   **B.** true   **C.** false   **D.** true   **E.** true

Increase in oxygen consumption in the tissues is known as the calorigenic action of thyroxine.

Thyroxine increases absorption of carbohydrate from the intestine but does not regulate gastrointestinal hormone secretion.

Fundamentals of Surgical Practice Chapter 14.

A 4. **A.** false   **B.** true   **C.** true   **D.** false   **E.** true

The rapid onset of a painful neck swelling is more suggestive of a thyroid cyst rather than a thyroid malignancy.

Advanced thyroid malignancy may result in swallowing difficulties.

Voice changes may suggest malignancy, particularly if the patient has developed a recurrent nerve palsy with easy breathlessness, air escape on speaking or bovine cough.

Fundamentals of Surgical Practice Chapter 14.

A 5. **A.** false   **B.** true   **C.** false   **D.** false   **E.** true

Tachycardia is a feature of hyperthyroidism.

Increased appetite is associated with hyperthyroidism.

Weight loss is more commonly a feature of hyperthyroidism.

Fundamentals of Surgical Practice Chapter 14.

A 6. **A.** false   **B.** true   **C.** true   **D.** false   **E.** true

Medical treatment of primary thyrotoxicosis may require carbimazole.

Radioiodine may be administered as a tailored dose to try and render the patient euthyroid. Long-term studies indicate that patients have a tendency to hypothyroidism as early as 10 years following therapy and therefore require long-term follow up. Alternatively, radioiodine can be administered as an ablating dose with all patients then commenced on thyroxine. No further follow up is required once the patient is stabilised on the replacement dose.

Propylthiouracil is an alternative medical therapy for thyrotoxicosis.

Thyroid lobectomy is an inadequate procedure for primary hyperthyroidism. Surgery should involve a bilateral subtotal thyroidectomy. A thyroid remnant of no more than 6 g should be left. Remnants larger than this are associated with a small incidence of recurrent thyrotoxicosis. The patient must be rendered euthyroid prior to surgery with anti-thyroid drugs or iodate. Some centres now advocate a near total thyroidectomy for thyrotoxicosis and turning all patients to a euthyroid state with thyroxine replacement. However, the long term sequelae, especially hypoparathyroidism, may not justify this more aggressive approach.

Thyroxine may be used as replacement therapy following ablative radioiodine therapy or near total thyroidectomy.

Fundamentals of Surgical Practice Chapter 14.

A 7. **A.** false **B.** true **C.** true **D.** true **E.** false

Hypocalcaemia is a complication associated with thyroidectomy due to manipulation or removal of parathyroid tissue.

Reactionary haemorrhage may result in rapid swelling within the neck tissue requiring immediate decompression.

Some patients may require replacement thyroxine treatment.

Fundamentals of Surgical Practice Chapter 14.

A 8. **A.** true **B.** true **C.** false **D.** true **E.** false

Pregnancy is a physiological cause of diffuse non-toxic goitre.

Thyroiditis is a common cause of diffuse non-toxic goitre but laryngitis does not cause goitre.

Fundamentals of Surgical Practice Chapter 14.

A 9. **A.** false **B.** true **C.** false **D.** true **E.** true

Hyperthyroidism is an indication for surgery in patients with multinodular goitre.

Multinodular goitre alone is not an indication for treatment but an increase in a dominant nodule, or a progressive enlargement of the entire gland are indications for surgical intervention.

Fundamentals of Surgical Practice Chapter 14.

A 10. **A.** false **B.** true **C.** true **D.** false **E.** true

70% of solitary thyroid nodules are due to adenomas. Approximately 20% are due to malignancy and 10% are due to cysts.

Since the cytology of follicular carcinoma and follicular adenoma is identical, it is impossible to exclude malignancy on a FNA of a follicular adenoma.

Since papillary carcinoma is frequently multifocal within the thyroid, total thyroidectomy is recommended followed by thyroxine to suppress TSH secretion.

Secondary spread of malignancy to the thyroid is rare, however hypernephromas are the most likely site of primary disease.

Fundamentals of Surgical Practice Chapter 14.

A 11. **A.** false **B.** true **C.** true **D.** false **E.** true

It is rarely possible to treat thyroid lymphoma surgically and the majority of patients are treated by external radiotherapy. The tumour tends to occur in the elderly and is rapidly progressive with a low 5-year survival rate.

Medullary carcinoma can occur as part of the multiple endocrine neoplasia (MEN) syndrome. Hyperparathyroidism is the commonest abnormality associated with MEN.

Papillary carcinoma tends to occur under the age of 40 years and is the commonest thyroid tumour in teenagers. At this age it is usually of a pure form histologically and responds well to treatment resulting in normal life expectancy.

Follicular carcinoma occurs most commonly in middle aged female patients. It is not associated with the good prognosis of papillary carcinoma; 5-year survival rate is approximately 50%.

Fundamentals of Surgical Practice Chapter 14.

A 12. **A.** false **B.** false **C.** true **D.** true **E.** true

The adrenal medulla produces noradrenaline and adrenaline, whereas the adrenal cortex secretes steroids, predominantly glucocorticoids, mineralocorticoids and sex hormones.

Cortisol and cortisone are powerful glucocorticoids.

Catecholamine release is stimulated by the sympathetic nervous system resulting in release directly into the inferior vena cava and immediately to the heart to exert an effect on the cardiovascular system. They dilate the pupil, increase the heart rate, raise blood pressure and blood sugar and lower the threshold in the reticular formation reinforcing the state of arousal.

ACTH release from the anterior pituitary gland controls the formation of glucocorticoids.

Fundamentals of Surgical Practice Chapter 14.

A 13. **A.** false **B.** true **C.** true **D.** true **E.** false

Cushing's disease is the excess production of glucocorticoids secondary to over stimulation of the adrenal cortex by a pituitary tumour. Clinically, patients present with hypertension.

A pituitary ACTH producing tumour tends to produce skin pigmentation as ACTH has a similar molecular structure to melanocyte stimulating hormone (MSH).

Moon face and buffalo hump are clinical features associated with Cushing's disease.

Fundamentals of Surgical Practice Chapter 14.

A 14. A. true   **B.** false   **C.** true   **D.** true   **E.** false

Primary hyperaldosteronism (Conn's syndrome) is most commonly due to an adrenal adenoma.

The main difference between primary and secondary hyperaldersteronism is regarding the plasma renin level. If this is low, primary disease is suggested and if it is high, the possibility of primary hyperaldosteronism can be eliminated.

In patients with malignant hypertension or with hypertension secondary to renal vascular disease, the reduced perfusion through the kidney will result in increased renin production resulting in secondary hyperaldosteronism. In Conn's syndrome, the patient develops elevated body sodium resulting in hypertension.

Conn's syndrome patients may have elevated plasma sodium level associated with hypokalaemia and alkalosis. Hyperaldosteronism results in the exchange of sodium for potassium and hydrogen, causing sodium retention and potassium loss. Therefore patients may have hypokalaemia.

Fundamentals of Surgical Practice Chapter 14.

A 15. A. true   **B.** false   **C.** false   **D.** true   **E.** true

Parathormone increases serum calcium.

Parathormone increases phosphate excretion in the urine.

Prolonged hypomagnesaemia increases parathormone secretion and may be associated with hypocalcaemia.

Fundamentals of Surgical Practice Chapter 14.

A 16. A. true   **B.** true   **C.** true   **D.** true   **E.** false

Over 90% of insulinomas are benign.

Whipple's triad is present in most patients with insulinoma. The features are a) symptoms precipitated by fasting b) significant hypoglycaemia during symptomatic episodes and c) relief of symptoms by glucose.

Localisation of insulinomas can be difficult. CT scanning is unreliable. Angiography, especially digital subtraction angiography is only accurate in 50% of cases. Percutaneous trans-hepatic catheterisation of the splenic vein with serial venous sampling along the line of the vein for insulin assay appears to be the most accurate technique, however, many patients proceed to open surgical exploration without the tumour being identified and localised pre-operatively.

As most insulinoma tumours are benign they can be treated surgically by enucleation and do not require radical resection techniques.

Gastrinoma is associated with the Zollinger-Ellison syndrome.

Fundamentals of Surgical Practice Chapter 14.

[A] **17.** **A.** false **B.** false **C.** false **D.** true **E.** true

Most carcinoid tumours arise in the appendix and distal small intestine but may occur in association with the duodenum or other parts of the gastrointestinal tract.

Carcinoid tumours are usually detected because of local effects rather than symptoms due to endocrine secretion.

Metastatic spread to the liver occurs in approximately 10% of patients resulting in the carcinoid syndrome. This consists of flushing, diarrhoea, bronchial constriction and right-sided cardiac valve disease.

Management of carcinoid tumours often involves resection of the primary tumour. Hepatic metastases may be treated by embolisation of the hepatic artery as these secondaries commonly appear to be totally dependent on the arterial circulation of the liver rather than the portal venous circulation. Debulking liver surgery may be beneficial in patients with advanced hepatic metastases to improve symptoms due to the carcinoid syndrome.

Fundamentals of Surgical Practice Chapter 14.

A 1.   **A.** true   **B.** false   **C.** false   **D.** true   **E.** false

Mammography is most useful when the breasts contain little dense glandular tissue and are composed predominantly of fat as in elderly female patients.

Microcalcification can be seen in both benign and malignant breast lesions.

Cytological examination of non-palpable lesions can be performed either stereotactically using mammographic-guided FNA or by ultrasound-guided FNA.

Triple assessment employs clinical examination, imaging (mammography, ultrasound) and FNAC and should achieve results with a sensitivity and specificity of >95%.

Excisional breast biopsy should be performed using a circumferential incision (using Langer's lines).

Fundamentals of Surgical Practice   Chapter 15.

A 2.   **A.** false   **B.** true   **C.** true   **D.** false   **E.** true

Blood-stained nipple discharge may be due to several causes, such as mammary duct ectasia, intraductal papilloma and occasionally during pregnancy.

Mondor's disease is characterised by thrombophlebitis of the superficial veins of the breast.

If discharge is from a single duct, then microdochectomy may be required.

Fundamentals of Surgical Practice   Chapter 15.

A. true   **B.** false   **C.** true   **D.** false   **E.** false

Mammary duct ectasia is one of the commonest causes of nipple inversion.

Paget's disease is characterised by reddening, excoriation and/or scaling of the skin of the nipple.

Congenital nipple inversion occurs in up to 20% of females.

Fundamentals of Surgical Practice Chapter 15.

A 4.   **A.** true   **B.** true   **C.** true   **D.** false   **E.** false

Breast pain can be treated with gamma-Linolenic acid with minimal side effects, although many patients simply require reassurance.

Non-cyclical mastalgia (breast pain) may arise from the musculoskeletal system (e.g. Tietz's syndrome – pain from the costochondral areas).

Diuretics have not been shown to be beneficial in the management of breast pain in randomised controlled trials.

Occasionally, total mastectomy (with or without breast reconstruction) may be indicated for refractory breast pain, but there is no role for limited resection of painful areas of breast tissue.

Fundamentals of Surgical Practice Chapter 15.

A 5.   **A.** false   **B.** false   **C.** false   **D.** false   **E.** true

Histological examination of mammary duct ectasia shows there is dilatation of ducts filled with inspissated breast secretions and lipid-filled macrophages.

The usual presenting feature is nipple discharge, however, nipple retraction may also occur.

Surgical treatment involves excision of all the major ducts as multiple ducts are likely to be involved and therefore not excision of a single duct (microdochectomy).

Fundamentals of Surgical Practice Chapter 15.

Breast

Answers

A 6. **A.** false **B.** true **C.** true **D.** true **E.** false

Sclerosing adenosis is characterised by prominent intralobular fibrosis and proliferation of small ductules or acini.

Epitheliosis is characterised by hyperplasia of the epithelium lining the terminal ducts and acini.

Numerous cysts (macro or micro) may develop in mammary dysplasia.

Fat necrosis may occur following trauma to the breast but is not associated with mammary dysplasia.

Fundamentals of Surgical Practice Chapter 15.

A 7. **A.** false **B.** true **C.** true **D.** true **E.** true

Gynaecomastia is associated with chronic liver failure, but not acute liver failure.

Approximately 25% of cases of gynaecomastia occur at the time of puberty and a further 25% of cases are idiopathic with no underlying cause being demonstrated.

Fundamentals of Surgical Practice Chapter 15.

A 8. **A.** false **B.** false **C.** false **D.** true **E.** true

Mammography in young women (<35 years) is difficult due to the density of the breast tissue and ultrasonography may provide more information.

The mammographic appearance of fat necrosis is similar to that of a breast carcinoma. Fine needle aspiration cytology should provide the diagnosis.

Small fibroadenomas in young women need not be excised provided the diagnosis is confirmed by FNAC.

Ultrasonography is useful to demonstrate the cystic nature of breast cysts which may be difficult to differentiate from fibroadenomas on mammography.

Fundamentals of Surgical Practice Chapter 15.

off

Breast

Answers

A. false   **B.** false   **C.** false   **D.** false   **E.** false

Early menarche is a known risk factor for breast carcinoma. The most important prognostic factor is the patient's lymph node status.

Lobular carcinoma is more commonly multifocal than ductal carcinoma.

With a thorough axillary clearance, no further treatment of the axilla is required, irrespective of whether there is involvement of the lymph nodes by tumour. Axillary radiotherapy following a clearance is associated with a significant incidence of lymphoedema (30%) and only a minimal improvement in regional disease control.

The greatest effect of Tamoxifen is seen in postmenopausal women and in those whose tumours are oestrogen-receptor positive.

Fundamentals of Surgical Practice Chapter 15.

A. false   **B.** false   **C.** false   **D.** true   **E.** false

A breast cancer staging of T2 N2 M1 indicates a tumour of >2 cm but <5 cm in diameter. If the tumour is fixed to the chest wall it is classified as T4.

N2 implies the ipsilateral axillary nodes are fixed. N3 implies involvement of the ipsilateral internal mammary lymph nodes. Paget's disease is classsified as Tis.

Fundamentals of Surgical Practice Chapter 15.

Thoracic Surgery   Answers

A 1.   **A.** false   **B.** false   **C.** false   **D.** false   **E.** false

A pneumothorax may occur spontaneously, particularly in tall thin patients. If this becomes a recurrent problem the patient may require a pleurodesis.

A pneumothorax does not always require intercostal tube drainage. If it is small it may be treated by needle aspiration.

A pneumothorax commonly occurs if air enters the pleural space from the lung or the exterior but it can also occur if air enters the pleural space from a ruptured oesophagus.

A chest drain should be inserted in the 5th intercostal space in the mid-axillary line.

A chest drain should be inserted above the rib below rather than below the rib above in order to avoid the neuro-vascular bundle.

Fundamentals of Surgical Practice   Chapter 16.

A 2.   **A.** false   **B.** true   **C.** true   **D.** false   **E.** true

A collection of pus within a lung lobe or lobes is referred to as a lung abscess. An empyema refers to the presence of pus in the pleural cavity.

Following organisation and thickening of granulation tissue lining an empyema, fibrosis may result. Excision of this may be necessary (decortication).

Bronchiectasis most likely affects the lower lobes although all parts of the lung may be involved.

Bronchiectasis is generally treated by postural drainage and antibiotics but sometimes resection of an infected lobe or segment may be indicated if the disease is localised.

Fundamentals of Surgical Practice   Chapter 16.

A 3. **A.** true **B.** true **C.** false **D.** false **E.** false

Venous engorgement of the face secondary to lung carcinoma is usually due to mediastinal spread and occlusion of the superior vena cava.

A Cushinoid appearance may be due to the production of ACTH, for example, from an oat cell tumour.

Horner's syndrome occurs with an apical lesion (Pancoast tumour).

Men are affected more frequently than women with a ratio of 4:1.

The most frequent type of lung carcinoma is a squamous carcinoma

Fundamentals of Surgical Practice Chapter 16.

A 4. **A.** true **B.** false **C.** false **D.** false **E.** true

Rib fracture in an elderly patient may be associated with significant morbidity due to poor respiratory effort secondary to pain with subsequent chest infection and even mortality.

A flail chest results when a number of adjacent ribs are fractured in more than one place.

The majority of patients with thoracic trauma do not require a thoracotomy. It is only required in less than 15% of patients.

Rupture of the diaphragm may be diagnosed by the presence of bowel loops in the chest cavity on a chest X-ray.

Fundamentals of Surgical Practice Chapter 16.

A 1. **A.** false **B.** false **C.** true **D.** false **E.** false

Approximately 60% of adenocarcinomas of the kidney occur in men.

Chemotherapy is of limited benefit. Radical nephrectomy (removal of the kidney, adrenal and perinephric fat) is the treatment of choice if there is no evidence of metastases.

The tumour arises in the renal tubules and has a propensity for haematogenous spread to bone. It may be associated with a left sided varicocele due to the tendency for the tumour to grow into the renal vein, hence occluding the left testicular vein. On the right side, the testicular vein drains directly into the vena cava.

Fundamentals of Surgical Practice Chapter 17.

A 2. **A.** true **B.** true **C.** true **D.** true **E.** false

PUJ obstruction may cause intermittent obstruction, precipitated by large fluid intake. It is treated by pyeloplasty (e.g. Anderson-Hynes).

Most stones <5 mm will pass spontaneously. If not, the resulting hydronephrosis may be treated by percutaneous nephrostomy or retrograde placement of a ureteric stent. The stone may then be treated by Extracorporeal Shock Wave Lithotripsy (ESWL) if it can be manipulated back into the renal pelvis. If the stone is far enough down the ureter it may be removed or fragmented using a ureteroscope.

A stricture may follow ureteroscopy or ureteric damage at open surgery.

Fundamentals of Surgical Practice Chapter 17.

A **3.** **A.** true   **B.** false   **C.** true   **D.** false   **E.** false

Over 80% of transitional cell carcinomas present with haematuria. Intravesical chemotherapy and external radiotherapy are useful treatment options for bladder TCC.

Smoking is a significant aetiological factor.

Transitional cell carcinoma of the bladder may be treated by endoscopic resection and regular check cystoscopy.

Fundamentals of Surgical Practice Chapter 17.

A **4.** **A.** true   **B.** false   **C.** false   **D.** true   **E.** true

In females, urinary retention may be associated with multiple sclerosis.

Chronic retention is painless and often associated with overflow incontinence.

Normal transurethral endoscopic findings are indicative of a functional problem (detrusor bladder neck dyssynergia or detrusor sphincter dyssynergia).

Fundamentals of Surgical Practice Chapter 17.

A **5.** **A.** true   **B.** false   **C.** true   **D.** true   **E.** false

Hesitancy, poor stream and post micturitional dribbling form the classical triad of presentation for benign prostatic hyperplasia.

When treated by transurethral resection, sterility results due to retrograde ejaculation which occurs following resection of the internal sphincter.

Non-surgical treatment is by an alpha-blocker (e.g. indoramin) or by a 5 alpha-reductase inhibitor (e.g. finasteride).

Fundamentals of Surgical Practice Chapter 17.

A 6. **A.** false **B.** true **C.** true **D.** false **E.** true

Carcinoma of the prostate tends to present late and thus radical curative surgery (radical prostatectomy), although feasible, is not usually possible.

Prostate Specific Antigen (PSA) is a specific tumour marker for this condition. This can be normal in localised prostate cancer but is invariably raised in metastatic disease. Bony metastases are usually sclerotic and confined to the axial skeleton.

Hormone manipulation is a palliative option and involves testosterone deprivation, either by bilateral orchidectomy or by drugs (e.g. luteinising hormone releasing hormone (LHRH) analogue which blocks the release of LH from the pituitary gland and thus stops production of testicular testosterone). This is given by a monthly subcutaneous injection.

Fundamentals of Surgical Practice Chapter 17.

A 7. **A.** true **B.** false **C.** false **D.** false **E.** false

A hydrocele usually has no septae, unlike an epididymal cyst which usually has multiple septae.

Surgery (e.g. Jaboulay procedure) is required to provide long-term resolution.

Treatment involves ligation of the testicular veins, either in the inguinal canal or retroperitoneum. The latter may be performed endoscopically.

In a young man with an acute testicular swelling, surgical exploration should always be undertaken to exclude a torsion.

Fundamentals of Surgical Practice Chapter 17.

A 8. **A.** true **B.** true **C.** true **D.** false **E.** false

The peak incidence for teratoma and seminoma is between ages 20–35 and 25–40 years respectively.

Tumour markers such as serum alpha-feto protein and beta-human chorionic gonadotrophin are useful as a diagnostic aid, in staging, in determining prognosis, in determining response to treatment and in detecting recurrence. Seminoma is highly radiosensitive. Cisplatinum based chemotherapy is used to treat metastatic teratoma.

Fundamentals of Surgical Practice Chapter 17.

Genitourinary System

Answers

A 1.   **A.** false   **B.** true   **C.** true   **D.** false   **E.** false

Surgical excision is the primary treatment for basal cell carcinoma: a microscopic surgical margin of 1 mm should be achieved.

Basal cell carcinoma may present as an ulcer or plaque, but may also present as a nodule or a black pigmented lesion.

Basal cell carcinoma of the face occurs most commonly above the line between the angle of the mouth and the pinna.

Fundamentals of Surgical Practice Chapter 18.

A 2.   **A.** true   **B.** true   **C.** true   **D.** false   **E.** false

Surgery and radiotherapy are the principal treatment modalities for cancers of the head and neck.

Elevated levels of antibodies to Epstein-Barr virus are indicative of nasopharyngeal cancer.

The peak age incidence for melanoma is 20–45 years.

Fundamentals of Surgical Practice Chapter 18.

A 3.   **A.** true   **B.** false   **C.** false   **D.** false   **E.** true

Laryngoceles occur laterally and are usually bilateral.

Branchial cysts present at the anterior border of the sternomastoid, at the junction of the upper third and the lower two thirds.

Cystic hygroma presents at birth in the lateral aspect of the neck and may extend into the pectoral region and axilla.

Dermoid cysts are situated in the suprasternal notch.

Fundamentals of Surgical Practice Chapter 18.

A 4. **A.** true **B.** false **C.** true **D.** true **E.** false

A thyroglossal cyst moves up on protrusion of the tongue because of its attachment to the hyoid bone. It is prone to infection because it is lined with ciliated respiratory epithelium.

Fundamentals of Surgical Practice Chapter 18.

A 5. **A.** true **B.** false **C.** true **D.** true **E.** false

A 6. **A.** true **B.** true **C.** false **D.** false **E.** false

Approximately 10% of parotid gland tumours are malignant, as are 50% of submandibular gland tumours.

A Wharthin's tumour is a benign lesion also known as a papillary cystadenoma lymphomatosum. The other benign tumour is the pleomorphic salivary adenoma.

Mucoepidermoid tumours are the commonest malignancy.

Pleomorphic salivary adenomas have pseudopodia which extend deeply into the gland therefore, superficial parotidectomy is the treatment of choice. This may result in damage to the facial nerve. Fine-needle aspiration cytology (FNAC) may be used for diagnosis of parotid tumours.

Fundamentals of Surgical Practice Chapter 18.

A 7. **A.** true **B.** true **C.** true **D.** false **E.** true

Gustatory sweating after superficial parotidectomy is known as Frey's syndrome.

Sialorrhoea may occur after excision of the submandibular gland due to damage to the mandibular branch of the facial nerve. The incision should therefore be kept more than 2 fingerbreadths below the ramus of the mandible.

Exposure keratitis after parotid surgery occurs due to damage to the zygomatic branch of the facial nerve.

Horner's syndrome (ptosis, meiosis, anhydrosis, enophthalmos) occurs after damage to the stellate ganglion. This has not been described with total parotidectomy.

Shoulder drop and weakness of the deltopectoral girdle after radical lymph node dissection of the neck occurs due to damage to the spinal accessory nerve.

Fundamentals of Surgical Practice Chapter 18.

A 1.   **A.** false   **B.** true   **C.** false   **D.** false   **E.** false

Eye opening, verbal response and motor response are used in the Glasgow Coma Scale (GCS). Pupillary reflexes are not.

The GCS is used as a serial measurement to detect change (particularly deterioration) in the level of consciousness.

A GCS score of less than 6 simply indicates that the patient has a very significant depression of consciousness. This may be due to an intracranial cause (e.g. haematoma, oedema) or hypoxia and hypotension due to hypovolaemia.

Fundamentals of Surgical Practice   Chapter 19.

A 2.   **A.** false   **B.** false   **C.** true   **D.** true   **E.** true

Increased intracranial pressure may typically be associated with bradycardia.

Tachycardia and hypertension together constitute Cushing's response.

The cerebellar tonsils and medulla are forced downwards through the foramen magnum leading ultimately to loss of consciousness and decerebration.

Fundamentals of Surgical Practice   Chapter 19.

A 3.   **A.** false   **B.** true   **C.** true   **D.** true   **E.** false

Chronic subdural haematoma is seen in patients on long-term anticoagulation.

The classical presenting feature is fluctuating confusion and drowsiness. To distinguish between chronic subdural haematoma and stroke, a CT scan should always be performed.

Fundamentals of Surgical Practice Chapter 19.

A 4. **A.** false **B.** false **C.** false **D.** false **E.** false

An immediate skull X-ray contributes little in the early assessment and management phase. The appropriate X-rays in such a patient are those of the chest, cervical spine and pelvis.

The level of consciousness is the most important physical sign in terms of assessment of the head injury.

Intravenous dexamethasone infusion is not indicated in the immediate resuscitation phase but may be used later if investigations reveal that cerebral oedema and raised intracranial pressure are present.

Restlessness, confusion and aggression suggest that the patient is hypoxic.

Fundamentals of Surgical Practice Chapter 19.

A 5. **A.** false **B.** true **C.** false **D.** false **E.** false

While haematogenous spread is a recognised cause of cerebral abscess (e.g. from bronchiectasis or lung abscess), direct spread from the paranasal sinuses, the mastoid or the middle ear is the most common cause.

Roughly 50% of intracranial tumours are metastatic, most frequently arising in lung or breast.

Meningiomas frequently invade local vascular structures (e.g. saggital sinus) but do not often metastasise.

In an acute head injury, a unilateral, fixed, dilated pupil may be caused by cerebral oedema.

Fundamentals of Surgical Practice Chapter 19.

Musculoskeletal System

Answers

A 1. **A.** true **B.** true **C.** true **D.** true **E.** false

Good fracture healing requires a good supply to the fractured bone ends, absence of soft tissue between the fracture ends, close apposition of the fracture ends and good nutritional status of the patient.

Fractures generally heal better in younger patients.

A slight degree of mobility at the fracture ends may stimulate more bone formation but excessive mobility would also contribute to poor fracture healing.

Fundamentals of Surgical Practice Chapter 20.

A 2. **A.** true **B.** true **C.** true **D.** true **E.** true

Delayed union may be due to the presence of a significant gap between fracture ends or associated soft tissue interposition. It may be also due to other factors such as poor nutritional status, poor blood supply to the fracture ends and old age.

Non-union is usually due to poor local blood supply with minimal or no callus formation. Bone grafting is usually necessary to encourage healing. When non-union occurs a false joint (pseudoarthrosis) may occur. Mal-union is usually due to incorrect fracture reduction and stabilisation.

Fundamentals of Surgical Practice Chapter 20.

A 3. **A.** true **B.** false **C.** true **D.** false **E.** false

The best examples of fractures associated with avascular necrosis are femoral neck and scaphoid fractures.

Fundamentals of Surgical Practice Chapter 20.

A 4.   **A.** false   **B.** true   **C.** false   **D.** true   **E.** true

Acute osteomyelitis is usually caused by staphylococcus or streptococcus.

Acute septic arthritis is usually due to staphylococcus, streptococcus or pseudomonas.

Fundamentals of Surgical Practice   Chapter 20.

Paediatric Surgery   Answers

A 1. **A.** true **B.** true **C.** true **D.** true **E.** false

A proximal oesophageal atresia with a distal tracheo-oesophageal fistula accounts for 85% of cases.

Associated anomalies include vertebral, anorectal, cardiac, TOF and esophageal atresia, renal and limb (i.e. VACTERL).

If the oesophageal ends are too far apart, a cervical oesophagostomy and gastrostomy are performed; anastomosis may later be attempted after growth of the oesophagus. If this is still not feasible, oesophageal substitution, using colon or stomach will be necessary.

Fundamentals of Surgical Practice Chapter 21.

A 2. **A.** false **B.** true **C.** true **D.** true **E.** false

Simple measures such as upright posturing, thickened feeds, antacids, H_2 blockers and proton pump inhibitors usually resolve the reflux.

Gastro-oesophageal reflux may present with respiratory symptoms due to reflux into the tracheobronchial tree and may present with upper GI bleeding due to oesophagitis. Oesophageal stricture may also occur.

Surgery (Nissen fundoplication) has a key role in management and is indicated for persistent failure to thrive, stricture and unresponsive oesophagitis.

Fundamentals of Surgical Practice Chapter 21.

A 3. **A.** false **B.** true **C.** false **D.** true **E.** true

Pyloric atresia is treated by gastroduodenostomy.

About one third of children with duodenal atresia also have Downs syndrome. Meconium ileus occurs in approximately 10% of children with cystic fibrosis.

Bilious vomiting, abdominal distension and failure to pass meconium are the classical presenting features of neonatal intestinal obstruction.

Fundamentals of Surgical Practice Chapter 21.

A 4. **A.** true **B.** false **C.** false **D.** false **E.** false

Ultrasonography is the investigation of choice for equivocal cases of infantile pyloric stenosis.

Immediate/emergency laparotomy for pyloric stenosis is not appropriate. Surgical management begins with rehydration and correction of biochemical abnormalities.

The peak incidence of intussussception is at 5–9 months and over 80% occur before age 2 years. Ileo-caecal is the most frequent type of intussussception, followed by ileo-ileal and jejuno-jejunal.

Fundamentals of Surgical Practice Chapter 21.

A 5. **A.** true **B.** true **C.** false **D.** true **E.** false

In gastroschisis there is no peritoneal sac and eviscerated bowel is exposed to amniotic fluid during intrauterine life, the bowel becoming matted and shortened, with its walls inflamed, thickened and covered with fibrin. In exomphalos there is a peritoneal sac and the bowel is relatively unaffected.

If primary fascial repair is not feasible, skin cover only may be achieved with later repair of the hernia or a prosthetic sheet may be used.

Three types of biliary atresia are recognised:

1. Atresia of the common bile duct (10%).
2. Atresia of the common hepatic duct (2%).
3. Atresia of most of or the entire extrahepatic duct system (88%).

Clearance of jaundice can be achieved using the Kasai operation in 50–60% of infants but there are often ongoing problems with cholangitis, portal hypertension and liver failure and 50–60% ultimately require liver transplantation.

Choledochal cyst should be excised and a hepaticojejunostomy used to establish biliary-enteric continuity. Cyst drainage into a jejunal loop is associated with a high incidence of anastomotic stricture, recurrent cholangitis, gallstones and an increased risk of malignancy.

Fundamentals of Surgical Practice Chapter 21.

A 6. **A.** false **B.** false **C.** true **D.** true **E.** false

Inguinal hernia is treated by herniotomy.

Hydrocele in a child is treated by ligation of the processus vaginalis similar to herniotomy.

Undescended testes affect 1–2% of boys. Orchidopexy is the recommended treatment for undescended testes, preferably between 1 and 2 years old.

Fundamentals of Surgical Practice Chapter 21.

Paediatric Surgery

Answers

Section 2

Extended Matching Questions (EMQs)

Options: **A.** ASA 1
B. ASA 2
C. ASA 4
D. ASA 4E
E. ASA 5E

For each of the patients described below, select the single most appropriate classification from the above. Each option may be used once, more than once or not at all.

1. A 62 year old man with severe ischaemic heart disease, but currently haemodynamically stable, undergoing surgery for a leaking abdominal aortic aneurysm.
2. A 90 year old female with peritonitis secondary to a perforated duodenal ulcer who has a systolic blood pressure of 80 mmHg.
3. A 58 year old female with chronic obstructive airways disease, who leads a normal and active life, who is about to undergo a colectomy.

Answers

1. — D. i.e. a patient with a severe, life threatening systemic disorder who is undergoing a major emergency operation.
2. — E. i.e. a moribund patient who requires emergency surgery.
3. — B.

Options:
A. Intravenous crystalloids (3 litres) for 24 h before surgery
B. Enoxaparin 20 mg/day
C. Enoxaparin 20 mg/TID
D. Intravenous cefuroxime 1.5 g plus metronidazole 500 mg
E. Intravenous cefuroxime 1.5 g

For each of the patients described below, select the single most appropriate answer from the above. Each option may be used once, more than once or not at all.

1. A 54 year old lady with obstructive jaundice who is due to undergo a hepaticojejunostomy.
2. A 60 year old gentleman who requires DVT prophylaxis during a sigmoid colectomy.
3. A 75 year old lady who requires antibiotic prophylaxis for a gastrectomy.
4. A 70 year old man who requires antibiotic prophylaxis during a right hemicolectomy.

Answers

1. — **A.** This is known as preoperative volume loading and is used as prophylaxis against potential extracellular fluid depletion and consequent renal impairment in patients with obstructive jaundice. This patient also requires antibiotic prophylaxis with intravenous cefuroxime and DVT prophylaxis with enoxaparin 20 mg.

2. — **B.** A single daily dose only is required for DVT prophylaxis. A TID regimen is used for treatment of DVT.

3. — **E.** Cefuroxime only is sufficient as anaerobes do not normally colonise the upper GI tract.

4. — **D.** These are the standard agents used in lower GI surgery.

Options: **A.** Continue
B. Discontinue

For each of the patients described below, select the single most appropriate answer from the above. Each option may be used once, more than once or not at all.

1. A 26 year old female taking a progesterone-only contraceptive pill who is to undergo a laparoscopic cholecystectomy.
2. A 65 year old man on warfarin who is to undergo a hemicolectomy.
3. A 35 year old female taking a combination oestrogen-progesterone pill who is to undergo day-case varicose vein ligation.
4. A 30 year old man with Crohn's disease who is taking 40 mg prednisolone per day and is due to undergo an ileal resection.
5. A 50 year old lady who is taking bendrofluazide for hypertension and is due to undergo a cholecystectomy.

Answers

1. — A. This pill poses no documented problems during surgery.
2. — B. The patient should be given enoxaparin 20 mg TID as an alternative.
3. — A. Patients undergoing day-case varicose vein surgery do not need to stop this type of pill but it should be stopped for 6 weeks prior to major abdominal surgery.
4. — A. Stopping this abruptly results in a risk of an adrenal crisis during surgery due to adrenocortical suppression. The surgery period should be covered with IV hydrocortisone.
5. — A. Antihypertensives should be continued up to the time of surgery.

Options: **A.** General anaesthesia
B. Spinal anaesthesia
C. Local anaesthesia
D. Regional nerve block
E. Epidural anaesthesia

For each of the patients described below, select the single most appropriate answer from the above. Each option may be used once, more than once or not at all.

1. A 75 year old man with chronic obstructive airways disease who is to undergo a hernia repair.
2. A patient who requires pain control following an AP resection of the rectum.
3. A 14 year old boy who requires wedge resection of a toenail.
4. A 50 year old man who requires pain control after a haemorrhoidectomy.

Answers

1. — B. Local anaesthetic may also be used.
2. — E. Major abdominal surgery should now rarely be contemplated without an 'epidural' for postoperative pain control.
3. — D. A ring block at the base of the toe is used. Local anaesthetic is not appropriate.
4. — D. A caudal block is used. Alternatively, long-acting local anaesthetic may be used.

Options: **A.** Haemolytic reaction
B. Iron overload
C. Febrile non-haemolytic reaction
D. Post-transfusion purpura
E. Hypocalcaemia
F. Graft-versus-host reaction

For each of the transfusion situations described below, select the most likely resulting complication.

1. A massive transfusion of cold blood.
2. A transfusion of blood to a patient who has become sensitized to leucocyte antigens by previous blood transfusions.
3. The inadvertent transfusion of ABO incompatible blood.

Answers

1. — E.
2. — C.
3. — A.

Options: **A.** Topical analgesia
             B. Local infiltration
             C. Nerve block
             D. Intravenous regional anaesthesia
             E. General anaesthesia
             F. Epidural analgesia

For each of the scenarios described below, select the most appropriate form of anaesthesia/analgesia.

1. A 67 year old man with Child-Pugh grade C alcoholic cirrhosis presents with a significant haematemesis. He is hypotensive (BP 85/50) and has a tachycardia (P 110 bpm). Following resuscitation he requires emergency upper gastrointestinal endoscopy.
2. A 72 year old lady with known ischaemic heart disease and COAD presents with a Colles fracture which requires manipulation. She has poor peripheral access.
3. An 85 year old man who is 6 weeks following a myocardial infarction presents with a strangulated inguinal hernia. He requires surgical intervention.
4. A 63 year old smoker has fallen 30 feet from a rooftop and has sustained a fractured right clavicle and fractures of ribs 5, 6, 7 and 8 on the left side. There is clinical evidence of a flail segment.

Answers

1. — E. Control of the airway is best achieved by performing OGD under general anaesthesia.
2. — B. In view of the significant comorbid medical condition of this patient, manipulation should be performed after local infiltration of anaesthetic agent into the fracture haematoma. A Bier's block (intravenous regional anaesthesia) is a useful alternative but may be difficult in this patient due to poor venous access.

3. — C. In view of recent myocardial infarct a general anaesthetic should be avoided. Groin hernia repair can be performed using a nerve block to achieve anaesthesia in the distribution of the ilioinguinal and iliohypogastric nerves.

4. — F. This man is at significant risk of developing respiratory complications and therefore an epidural for pain relief combined with intensive physiotherapy may prevent the development of subsequent complications.

Options: **A.** Clean wound
B. Potentially contaminated wound
C. Contaminated wound
D. Dirty wound

For each of the surgical procedures below, select the most appropriate classification of wound.

1. Laparoscopic cholecystectomy. *B*
2. Pilonidal abscess. *D*
3. Thyroid lobectomy. *A*
4. Laparotomy for perforated duodenal ulcer. *D*
5. Femoral hernia repair. *A*
6. Tracheostomy. *A*
7. Laparotomy for perforated diverticular disease. *D*

Answers

1. — **B.**
2. — **D.**
3. — **A.**
4. — **D.**
5. — **A.**
6. — **A.**
7. — **D.**

Wound Closure | Theme 8

Options: **A.** Primary closure
B. Delayed primary closure
C. Closure by secondary intention
D. Escharotomy
E. Excision and skin grafting

For each of the surgical procedures described, select the most appropriate method of wound management.

1. Full thickness burn to face.
2. Epigastric hernia repair.
3. Perianal abscess incision.
4. Circumferential burns to chest.
5. Gunshot wound to thigh.

Answers

1. — E. Excision and skin grafting will minimise scarring.
2. — A.
3. — C. Wound is packed with paraffin ribbon gauze and allowed to heal by secondary intention.
4. — D. Circumferential burns to chest will restrict chest expansion and therefore escharotomy is performed to maintain respiratory function.
5. — C. Wound is debrided and left to heal by secondary intention.

Options:
- **A.** Chest X-ray
- **B.** CT scan
- **C.** 16-lead ECG
- **D.** Blind immediate burr holes
- **E.** Insertion of a central venous line for CVP monitoring
- **F.** Intraventricular catheter placement for intracranial pressure monitoring
- **G.** Transfer to a neurosurgical unit
- **H.** Endotracheal intubation and ventilation

For each of the clinical scenarios described, select the most likely initial management option.

1. A 19 year old motorcyclist involved in a road traffic accident who is comatose with a Glasgow Coma Scale of 6.
2. A 35 year old man with an open head wound and a depressed skull fracture.
3. A 45 year old mountaineer who has been hit on the head by a falling rock remains confused with a Glasgow Coma Scale of 13 after initial assessment and resuscitation.
4. A 13 year boy with a Glasgow Coma Scale of 14 but has persisting headache and vomiting after falling off his bicycle.

Answers

1. — **H.** The initial management in a patient with a GCS <8 is to secure the airway by endotracheal intubation and ventilation.
2. — **G.** This patient will require neurosurgical intervention.
3. — **B.** An intracranial haematoma must be excluded.
4. — **B.**

Options: A. Gram negative septicaemia
   B. Endotoxaemia
   C. Multiple organ dysfunction syndrome (MODS)
   D. Bacteraemia
   E. Systemic inflammatory response syndrome (SIRS)
   F. Sepsis
   G. Adult respiratory distress syndrome (ARDS)
   H. Infection

For each of the definitions listed below, select the most accurate term.

1. The clinical syndrome of systemic inflammation resulting from invasive infection.
2. The presence of viable bacteria in the bloodstream.
3. A clinical syndrome characterised by 2 or more of the following criteria: Temperature >38°C or <36°C; heart rate >90 bpm; respiratory rate >20 or PaCO$_2$ <32 mmHg; WBC >12 or <4.
4. Sepsis associated with respiratory failure, renal failure, hepatic dysfunction and coagulopathy.

Answers

1. — F. Infection may invoke a systemic host response and this is known as sepsis.
2. — D.
3. — E. The diagnostic criteria reported by the American College of Chest Physicians/Society of Critical Care Medicine Consensus Conference.
4. — C.

Options: **A.** Sensitivity
B. Specificity
C. Cross-sectional study
D. Case-controlled study
E. Cohort study

For each of the definitions described below, select the single most appropriate answer from the above. Each option may be used once, more than once or not at all.

1. The number of true positives which are correctly defined by the test. *A*
2. The number of true negatives which are defined by the test. *B*
3. A study in which a group of subjects is identified and then followed *E* up long-term.
4. A study in which a patient with a given condition is compared with one or more controls, matched as far as possible for characteristics *D* other than the disease under investigation.
5. A study in which data is collected at a single point in time with *C* subjects being contacted only once.

Answers

1. — A.
2. — B.
3. — E.
4. — D.
5. — C.

Options: **A.** Systemic lupus erythematosus
B. Myasthenia gravis
C. Rheumatoid arthritis
D. Idiopathic thrombocytopenic purpura (ITP)
E. Grave's disease
F. Hashimoto's thyroiditis
G. Auto-immune haemolytic anaemia

For each of the patients described below, select the single most appropriate answer from the above. Each option may be used once, more than once, or not at all.

1. A 60 year old female patient with goitre and features of hyperparathyroidism who is currently being treated with radioactive iodine.
2. A patient with a previous thymectomy who is currently being treated with steroids.
3. A child who suffers from recurrent spontaneous bleeding which was ultimately treated by splenectomy.
4. A 50 year old female with elevated antibodies to Thyroglobulin who has a hard goitre and is currently being treated with steroids and thyroxine.
5. A middle aged female patient with a skin rash, arthritis and renal failure.
6. A patient who develops anaemia and who has a history of drug ingestion (e.g. penicillin).

Answers

1. — E.
2. — B.
3. — D.
4. — F.
5. — A.
6. — G.

Intestinal Obstruction

Theme 13

Options:
- **A.** Extended right hemicolectomy
- **B.** Adhsiolysis
- **C.** Hartman's procedure
- **D.** Subtotal colectomy and ileorectal anastomosis
- **E.** Three-stage approach with defunctioning colostomy, colonic resection and closure of colostomy
- **F.** Intestinal stenting with an expandable metallic stent
- **G.** Colonoscopic decompression

For each of the clinical scenarios described below, select the most suitable therapeutic procedure.

1. An 80 year old lady with an obstructing neoplastic lesion in the transverse colon.
2. An 85 year old lady who develops gross abdominal distension 4 days following insertion of a dynamic hip screw for a fractured neck of femur.
3. A 91 year man with congestive heart failure and chronic obstructive airways disease is found to have an obstructing rectal tumour with liver metastases.
4. A 35 year old man with central colicky abdominal pain has dilated loops of small bowel on an abdominal X-ray. He had undergone appendicectomy as a child.
5. A 70 year old man has gross distension of his caecum, ascending, transverse and descending colon on abdominal X-ray and has complete obstruction in the distal sigmoid colon on an unprepared barium enema.

Answers

1. — A. An extended right hemicolectomy is the procedure of choice for a malignant lesion in the distal transverse colon.

2. — G. Colonic pseudo-obstruction may occur following internal fixation of a fractured neck of femur. Barium enema can confirm the diagnosis of pseudo-obstruction and colonoscopic decompression is usually effective.

3. — F. Intestinal stenting with an expandable metallic stent is a minimal technique which should provide effective palliation for this patient avoiding surgical intervention.

4. — B. A band adhesion is the common cause of small bowel obstruction if the patient has had a previous abdominal procedure.

5. — D. Gross distension of the proximal large bowel will invariably indicate compromised blood supply and therefore a subtotal colectomy with ileorectal anastomosis would be preferable to a colo-colonic anastomosis.

Intestinal Obstruction

Theme 13

Options: **A.** Abdominal ultrasound
B. CT scan of abdomen
C. Barium enema
D. Upper gastrointestinal endoscopy
E. ERCP

For each of the clinical scenarios described, select the most appropriate investigation.

1. A 42 year old lady with known gallstones presents with a two week history of jaundice.
2. A 78 year old man with a history of dysphagia and weight loss.
3. A 50 year old man with a known history of chronic pancreatitis who presents with exacerbation of his pain and on examination has a fullness in his upper abdomen.
4. A 46 year old man presents with gallstone induced severe acute pancreatitis with abnormal liver function tests.
5. An 84 year old lady with gross abdominal distension 3 days following internal fixation of a fractured neck of femur.

Answers

1. — E. The most likely diagnosis is obstruction of the extrahepatic biliary tree by a ductal calculi.
2. — D. The most likely diagnosis is of a malignant stricture of the oesophagus.
3. — B. This man may have developed a pancreatic pseudocyst as a recognised complication of chronic pancreatitis. CT scanning may confirm the diagnosis and provide helpful information as to the most appropriate management option, i.e. endoscopic or surgical drainage procedure.
4. — E. Early ERCP has been shown to improve the outcome for patients with predicted severe acute gallstone-related pancreatitis if performed within 48 h of disease onset.
5. — C. The likely diagnosis is large bowel pseudo-obstruction, however, mechanical obstruction must be excluded by means of a barium enema.

Perianal Conditions Theme 15

Options:
  A. Anal fissure
  B. Anal fistula
  C. Perianal haematoma
  D. Pilonidal sinus
  E. Perianal abscess
  F. Prolapsed thrombosed haemorrhoid
  G. Proctalgia fugax

For each of the clinical scenarios described below, select the most likely diagnosis.

1. A 20 year old female complains of severe pain after defaecation and notes some bright red blood on the toilet paper.
2. A 30 year old man complains of a painful swelling at the anus following an episode of straining at stool. A tender subcutaneous swelling resembling a blackcurrant is visualised.
3. A 24 year old man complains of pain, bleeding and discharge from a midline opening 6 cm posterior to the anus in the natal cleft.
4. A 45 year old man complains of intermittent discharge of foul-smelling fluid from an indurated area lateral to the anus. Examination reveals a small pit in this region.

Answers

1. — A. Severe pain following defaecation is a feature of anal fissures.
2. — C. This is the classical presentation and findings associated with a perianal haematoma.
3. — D. A pilonidal sinus commonly opens in the midline in the natal cleft but may also have lateral openings and subcutaneous tracts.
4. — B. An anal fistula frequently presents in this way and insertion of a probe should identify the communication with the bowel.

Options: **A.** Atheroma
             B. Aneurysm
             C. Diabetes
             D. Buerger's disease
             E. Takayasu's disease
             F. Bechet's disease
             G. Infection

For each of the patients described below, select the single most appropriate answer from the above. Each option may be used once, more than once or not at all.

1. A chronic arteritis typically affecting young adult male smokers and characterised by inflammation involving small and medium sized arteries and the adjacent vein.
2. A chronic arteritis affecting mainly young women and children and typically involving the aorta and its branches.
3. A microangiopathy occurs in this condition and compounds the problems caused by the already increased risk of atherosclerosis.
4. A chronic degenerative condition involving deposits in the arterial intima, which consist of calcium, fibrous tissue, lipids, carbohydrates and blood products.

Answers

1. — D. This is the classical description of Buerger's disease.
2. — E.
3. — C.
4. — A.

Options: **A.** Thrombosis
B. Embolism
C. Raynaud's phenomenon

For each of the patients described below, select the single most appropriate answer from the above. Each option may be used once, more than once or not at all.

1. An 85 year old lady who is in atrial fibrillation presents with a cold, pulseless left leg.
2. A 70 year old man with chronic vascular insufficiency who recently underwent lower limb arterial surgery presents with a cold, painful leg.
3. A vasospastic condition which may present with severe acute peripheral ischaemia.

Answers

1. — B. This is the classical type of patient who may present with a distal embolus from the left atrium.
2. — A. The combination of atherosclerosis and recent surgery predispose to thrombosis.
3. — C.

Management of Vascular Disease

Theme 18

Options:
  A. Streptokinase
  B. Angioplasty
  C. Endarterectomy
  D. Surgical bypass
  E. Sympathectomy
  F. Amputation

For each of the patients described below, select the single most appropriate answer from the above. Each option may be used once, more than once or not at all.

1. A 60 year old female with a short segment stenosis of the internal carotid artery.   C
2. A 28 year old female with palmar hyperhidrosis.   E
3. A 68 year old man with a short segment stenosis of the distal femoral artery.   B
4. A 65 year old man who develops acute thrombosis following a femoral angioplasty.   A
5. A 70 year old man with intermittent claudication due to long segment occlusion of the distal femoral artery.   D
6. A 60 year old man with cutaneous ulceration secondary to extensive femoral and popliteal atherosclerosis.   E

Answers

1. — C.
2. — E. The endoscopic transthoracic route is most frequently used.
3. — B.
4. — A.
5. — D. A femoro-popliteal bypass is the appropriate procedure.
6. — E. This is one of the main indications for lower limb sympathectomy although it is rarely used. It should be remembered that it may increase claudication pain by diverting an already reduced blood flow to the skin.

Options: **A.** Mammary duct ectasia
B. Fibroadenoma
C. Breast cyst
D. Fibrocystic disease of the breast
E. Breast carcinoma
F. Paget's disease

For each of the clinical findings described below, select the most likely diagnosis.

1. A palpable hard breast lump with associated peau d'orange.   E
2. A scaly, erythematous nipple.   F
3. Intermittent painless green nipple discharge with no palpable breast   A
   abnormality and a normal mammogram.
4. A smooth, well-circumscribed, mobile lump in a 20 year old girl.   B
5. A solitary breast lump which is hypoechoeic on ultrasound examination.   C
6. A nodular area in the upper outer quadrant of the breast associated   D
   with cyclical breast pain.

Answers

1. — **E.** A hard breast lump with associated skin changes is a cancer
   until proven otherwise.
2. — **F.**
3. — **A.** Mammary duct ectasia may present with a discharge that varies
   in colour from clear to black and may be from one duct or
   multiple ducts. The discharge may contain blood and may be
   associated with nipple retraction.
4. — **B.** A fibroadenoma is frequently referred to as a 'breast mouse'
   due to its mobility.
5. — **C.** Aspiration usually reveals green-brown fluid and disappearance
   of the lump.
6. — **D.** Fibrocystic disease or mammary dysplasia arises as a result of a
   disordered proliferation and involution of breast tissues that
   occurs as part of the normal cyclical physiological process
   during the reproductive years.

Options **A.** Conservative management with observation
 B. Needle thoracocentesis
 C. Chest drain insertion
 D. Intercostal nerve block
 E. Thoracic epidural
 F. Thoracotomy

For each of the patients described below, select the single most appropriate answer from the above. Each option may be used once, more than once or not at all.

1. A 35 year old male who is involved in a road traffic accident and has sustained a fracture of the 8th rib on the left side.
2. An 85 year old female who fell downstairs and sustained fractures of the 4th, 5th, 6th and 7th ribs on the right side.
3. A 40 year old male who was stabbed in the left side of the chest and has sustained a 30% pneumothorax plus a small haemothorax.
4. A 16 year old girl who fell off her bicycle and has sustained a small (less than 10%) left sided pneumothorax.

Answers

1. — A. Such a patient does not need a chest drain or a nerve block.
2. — D. An elderly patient with such a large number of fractured ribs is at significant risk of poor inspiratory effort and atelectasis due to pain. Narcotic analgesia would further reduce inspiratory effort and pain relief is best given by intercostal nerve block or even by a thoracic epidural.
3. — C. Chest drain insertion is the appropriate treatment for such a patient – thoracotomy is not indicated and is only necessary in approximately 15% of chest trauma cases.
4. — B. Needle thoracocentesis is suitable for managing such a small pneumothorax but the patient should be closely monitored in case the pneumothorax increases.

Chest X-ray Findings

Theme 21

Options: **A.** Widening of the mediastinum
 B. Fractured ribs 3–8 on left hand side
 C. Fractured ribs 3–5, each in 2 places on the right hand side
 D. Shadow with air/fluid level superimposed on the heart shadow
 E. Gas filled loops of small bowel in left chest cavity

For each of the diagnoses below, select the single most appropriate answer from the above. Each option may be used once, more than once or not at all.

1. Rolling hiatus hernia.
2. Rupture of left hemi-diaphragm.
3. Flail chest.
4. Rupture of the ascending aorta.

Answers

1. — D. A rolling hiatus hernia is also known as a paroesophageal hernia and may produce a shadow with an air fluid level on chest X-ray. The more common sliding hiatus hernia does not produce such a sign.

2. — E.

3. — C. In order for a flail segment to occur one or more ribs must be fractured in more than one place.

4. — A.

Options: **A.** Testicular torsion
B. Epididymal cyst
C. Hydrocele
D. Epididymo-orchitis
E. Haematoma
F. Seminoma
G. Teratoma
H. Varicocele

For each of the scenarios described below, select the single most appropriate answer from the above. Each option may be used once, more than once or not at all.

1. A painless 2 cm diameter swelling at the upper pole of the testis *B* which transilluminates and is palpable separately from the testis.
2. A painless 8 cm swelling which transilluminates. The testis cannot be *C* palpated separately from it.
3. An acutely painful and tender testicular swelling in a 14 year old boy *A* with no history of trauma.
4. An enlarged, painful and tender testis in a 50 year old man. The *D* symptoms have been present for 2 weeks and there have been 2 previous episodes in the last year.
5. A painless, non-tender testicular swelling in a 27 year old associated *G.* with an elevated serum beta-HCG and alpha-feto protein.
6. A painless non-tender testicular swelling in a 45 year old with *F* enlarged para-aortic nodes on CT scan.

Answers

1. — B.
2. — C.
3. — A.
4. — D.
5. — G.
6. — F. Teratoma tends to occur in younger men (25–35) while seminoma tends to occur in those slightly older (30–45).

Treatment of Scrotal Swellings — Theme 23

Options: **A.** Antibiotics
B. Jaboulay procedure
C. Local excision
D. Immediate surgical exploration
E. Conservative management and analgesia
F. Left testicular vein ligation

For each of the patients described below, select the single most appropriate answer from the above. Each option may be used once, more than once or not at all.

1. A 45 year old with a 3 cm transilluminable swelling on the upper pole of the right testis which is causing him periodic pain.
2. A 30 year old with a 5 cm swelling around the left testis following a kick during a football game.
3. A 15 year old boy with a painful, tender right scrotal swelling of 8 h duration.
4. A 68 year old with a 15 cm transilluminable left scrotal swelling which causes significant discomfort.
5. A 28 year old with a vascular swelling around the left testis which increases in size on standing.

Answers

1. — **C.** This is the treatment for a symptomatic epididymal cyst.
2. — **E.** Such a scrotal haematoma should be treated conservatively.
3. — **D.** In such a situation antibiotics should not be the first treatment. Immediate exploration for a testicular torsion is mandatory.
4. — **B.** This is the appropriate procedure for a hydrocele.
5. — **E.** This is the appropriate treatment for a varicocele – it may be performed laparoscopically or via an oblique lateral abdominal incision. An ultrasound of the left kidney, to exclude a left hypernephroma growing into the left renal vein and hence occluding the left testicular vein, should be performed prior to surgery (on the right side, the testicular vein drains directly into the vena cava).

Options: **A.** Benign nodular hyperplasia (BNH) of the prostate
B. Carcinoma of the prostate
C. Pelvi-ureteric junction (PUJ) obstruction
D. Cystitis
E. Vesico-ureteric reflux (VUR)
F. Transitional cell carcinoma

For each of the patients described below, select the single most appropriate answer from the above. Each option may be used once, more than once or not at all.

1. A 28 year old female with intermittent right flank pain, precipitated by drinking large volumes of fluid.
2. A 48 year old female with frequency of micturition, pain on micturition and microscopic haematuria.
3. A 65 year old male with frequency, hesitancy, slow stream and post-micturition dribbling.
4. A 75 year old male with severe back pain, lethargy and weight loss.
5. A 60 year old smoker with painless haematuria.

Answers

1. — **C.** This is the typical presentation of PUJ obstruction.
2. — **D.**
3. — **A.** Very typical symptoms for BNH of the prostate.
4. — **B.** Don't forget to check the prostate specific antigen (PSA) in any older male patient presenting with back pain!
5. — **F.**

Options: **A.** Branchial cyst
B. Cystic hygroma
C. Thyroglossal cyst
D. Zenker's diverticulum
E. Dermoid cyst
F. Parotitis
G. Teratoma
H. Goitre
I. Malignant lymphadenopathy
J. Pleomorphic salivary adenoma of the parotid

For each of the scenarios described below, select the single most appropriate answer from the above. Each option may be used once, more than once or not at all.

1. A cystic swelling at the junction of the upper one third and lower two thirds of the sternomastoid muscle.
2. A midline cystic swelling which moves upwards on protrusion of the tongue.
3. A lateral diffuse swelling which moves upwards on swallowing.
4. A lateral neck swelling in a patient complaining of dysphagia and regurgitation of recently ingested food.
5. A firm non-tender swelling situated over the body of the mandible
6. A cystic swelling in the suprasternal notch.

Answers

1. — **A.** This is the classical site for a branchial cyst or sinus (at anterior border of sternomastoid).
2. — **C.**
3. — **H.**
4. — **D.**
5. — **J.**
6. — **E.** Other sites for dermoid cysts include the inner and outer canthus at the eye.

Depressed Level of Consciousness

Options:
A. Narcotisation
B. Extradural haematoma
C. Subdural haematoma
D. Subarachnoid haemorrhage
E. Intracerebral haematoma
F. Diffuse cerebral oedema
G. Depressed skull fracture

For each of the patients described below, select the single most appropriate answer from the above. Each option may be used once, more than once or not at all.

1. A 76 year old lady on warfarin for treatment of atrial fibrillation develops insidious confusion and drowsiness.   C

2. A 14 year old boy who fell off his bicycle and initially has a normal Glasgow Coma Scale develops a fairly rapid deterioration in his level of consciousness 3 h later in the observation ward.   B

3. A 72 year old lady develops shallow slow breathing and a progressive fall in oxygen saturation from 98% to 75%, in the postoperative period.   A

4. A 65 year old alcoholic male develops progressive confusion and drowsiness following a minor fall.   C

5. A 24 year old lady develops progressive depression of consciousness level several hours after an overdose of paracetamol.   F

Answers

1. — **C.** Subdural haematoma is a well recognised and significant complication of long-term anticoagulation.

2. — **B.** This is the classical scenario for an extradural haematoma. It typically presents several hours after an injury to the temporal region and is due to an expanding haematoma, secondary to rupture of the middle meningeal artery.

3. — **A.** This is the typical situation caused by excess administration of narcotic analgesics (e.g. morphine). It should be treated by

reversal of the narcotic agent using naloxone, oxygen therapy and ventilatory assistance (e.g. Ambu bag), if necessary.

4. — C. This is a relatively common cause of chronic subdural haematoma. It is treated by burr hole and aspiration. A typical brown/black fluid is obtained.

5. — F. Paracetamol overdose causes liver failure which subsequently results in diffuse cerebral oedema and unconsciousness.

Fracture Complications

Theme 27

Options:
- **A.** Avascular necrosis
- **B.** Volkman's ischaemic contracture
- **C.** Myositis ossificans
- **D.** Sudeck's atrophy
- **E.** Fat embolism

For each of the descriptions below, select the single most appropriate answer from the above. Each option may be used once, more than once or not at all.

1. The development of a swollen limb with shiny, smooth, mottled skin which may be excessively sweaty – it tends to occur following hand or wrist fractures.
2. Development of respiratory complications following major fractures e.g. femoral or pelvic fracture.
3. Necrosis of bone following a fracture where the blood supply to the bone is tenuous e.g. femoral neck or scaphoid.
4. Occurs as a result of an unrecognised compartment syndrome.
5. Development of bone formation in soft tissue and haematoma surrounding a fracture site.

Answers

1. — D.
2. — E.
3. — A.
4. — B.
5. — C.

Options:
- **A.** Duodenal atresia
- **B.** Annular pancreas
- **C.** Malrotation
- **D.** Small bowel atresia
- **E.** Intussussception
- **F.** Colonic atresia
- **G.** Meckel's diverticulum

For each of the patients described below, select the single most appropriate answer from the above. Each option may be used once, more than once or not at all.

1. A 6 month old child presents with severe abdominal pain, vomiting and rectal bleeding.   E

2. A neonate presents with bilious vomiting, abdominal distension and failure of passage of meconium.   D

3. A neonate presents with bilious vomiting and a 'double bubble' sign on a plain abdominal X-ray.   B

Answers

1. — E. This classical triad is present in only 30% of cases.

2. — D. The degree of abdominal distension depends on the level of the atresia. With more proximal jejunal atresia the distension will obviously be less.

3. — B. Bilious vomiting occurs only in post-ampullary lesions. The 'double bubble' sign is due to the distended stomach and first part of the duodenum.

Options: **A.** Exomphalos
B. Gastroschisis
C. Hypertrophic pyloric stenosis
D. Necrotising enterocolitis
E. Intussussception

For each of the patients described below, select the single most appropriate answer from the above. Each option may be used once, more than once or not at all.

1. A baby is born with intestinal loops outside the abdominal cavity, covered by a peritoneal sac.
2. A 3–4 week old baby develops non-bilious projectile vomiting.
3. A low birth weight infant develops lethargy, poor feeding, vomiting, abdominal distension and blood in the stool.

Answers

1. — A. In gastroschisis there is no peritoneal sac.
2. — C. The diagnosis is confirmed by ultrasound – treatment involves a pyloromyotomy.
3. — D.